"Most people love the feelings of belonging and acceptance that come with being a member of a group. What a better approach to help people of all ages make connections with others and learn more about themselves in the process! This timely book emphasizes the importance of group play therapy and the power of working together. The various authors present a wide variety of experiential group activities that serve a multitude of populations. You're sure to find activities to enhance your practice and learn more about Group Play Therapy!"

Scott Riviere, *MS, LPC, RPT-S, owner K.I.D.Z. Inc.*

"Wow! This book you have in your hands covers so much information about group play therapy. The book provides information about the basics of group play therapy: who, why, where, and how, along with an overview of important ethical considerations. AND there's more...the editors have gathered well-grounded authors who have demonstrated expertise in a plethora of approaches to group play therapy, and these authors have written fascinating chapters about a variety of applications of group play therapy, across a rich collection of settings and populations. If you want to work with clients using the modality of group play therapy, you need this book."

Terry Kottman, *PhD, RPT-S, LMHC, founder and director, League of Extraordinary Adlerian Play Therapists*

Implementing Play Therapy with Groups

Implementing Play Therapy with Groups is a new and innovative edited book bringing together experts from across the field of play therapy to explore how to facilitate group play therapy across challenging settings, diagnoses, and practice environments.

Applying theoretical and empirical information to address treatment challenges, each chapter focuses on a specific treatment issue and explores ways the reader can implement group work within their play therapy work. Chapters also provide contemporary evidence-based clinical information in providing group therapy with specific populations such as working with children who have been exposed to violence, trauma, adoption, foster care, those who are chronically medically fragile, and more.

This book will bring awareness to, and provide easily implemented play therapy knowledge and interventions for, child and family therapists who work in a range of settings including schools, hospitals, residential treatment centers, and community mental health settings.

Clair Mellenthin, LCSW, RPT-S, is an international speaker, author, and Registered Play Therapist Supervisor. Clair is the author of the bestselling book *Attachment Centered Play Therapy*. She is the director of Child & Adolescent Services at Wasatch Family Therapy in Utah.

Jessica Stone, PhD, is an international speaker, clinical supervisor, and registered play therapist. She is the co-creator of The Virtual Sandtray®© and the developer of Digital Play Therapy.™

Robert Jason Grant, EdD, is a Licensed Professional Counselor, Advanced Certified Autism Specialist, and is the creator of AutPlay® Therapy. He serves on the Board of Directors for the Association for Play Therapy and is an accomplished author, advocate, and trainer.

Implementing Play Therapy with Groups
Contemporary Issues in Practice

Edited by
Clair Mellenthin, Jessica Stone, and Robert Jason Grant

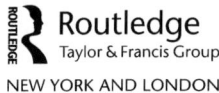

Routledge
Taylor & Francis Group

NEW YORK AND LONDON

Cover image: Getty Images

First published 2022
by Routledge
605 Third Avenue, New York, NY 10158

and by Routledge
2 Park Square, Milton Park, Abingdon, Oxon OX14 4RN

Routledge is an imprint of the Taylor & Francis Group, an informa business

Library of Congress Cataloging-in-Publication Data
Names: Mellenthin, Clair, editor. | Stone, Jessica (Child psychologist), editor. | Grant, Robert Jason, 1971- editor.
Title: Implementing play therapy with groups : contemporary issues in practice / edited by Clair Mellenthin, Jessica Stone, Robert Jason Grant.
Description: New York, NY : Routledge, 2022. | Includes bibliographical references and index. |
Identifiers: LCCN 2021025647 (print) | LCCN 2021025648 (ebook) | ISBN 9780367556587 (hardback) | ISBN 9780367556563 (paperback) | ISBN 9781003094531 (ebook)
Subjects: LCSH: Group play therapy.
Classification: LCC RJ505.P6 I47 2022 (print) | LCC RJ505.P6 (ebook) | DDC 618.92/891653--dc23
LC record available at https://lccn.loc.gov/2021025647
LC ebook record available at https://lccn.loc.gov/2021025648

ISBN: 978-0-367-55658-7 (hbk)
ISBN: 978-0-367-55656-3 (pbk)
ISBN: 978-1-003-09453-1 (ebk)

DOI: 10.4324/9781003094531

Typeset in Times New Roman
by Taylor & Francis Books

Contents

Illustrations

Figures

Tables

Foreword

Athena A. Drewes, PsyD, RPT-S

Play therapy as a treatment modality is growing in acceptance and use around the world. It is primarily used with children, teens, and families through individual treatment modalities and many clinicians are trained in and most comfortable with these individual modalities. However, children often find social situations in school and outside of the home difficult and anxiety provoking, and often lack social and relational skills, which cannot be addressed solely in individual therapy.

Consequently, group play therapy has often been the treatment of choice with a variety of populations and disorders. There are several benefits to group play therapy. Group play therapy allows for the efficient use of time, materials, and space in reaching more children (Ginott, 1961; Sweeney & Homeyer, 1999; Sweeney et al., 2014). It allows the child the opportunity to not only socialize with peers, but also to realize that they are not alone in their problems; that others share similar experiences, feelings, and fears. Often children will quickly feel safe with peers and can be more readily drawn into activities within the therapy room than they might experience within individual therapy. With peers in a group therapy setting, the children further benefit from role playing and modeling provided by interacting with the higher functioning children.

Within group play therapy, children can play out their feelings and experiences when words cannot be found or there is resistance to sharing deepest fears even in the most emotionally safe and caring of environments. They may feel safer in a group setting to reveal family and personal events. With peer support, play therapy interventions, and making treatment playful, the child can find nonverbal ways to communicate the pain and troubles held within. Having play approaches/interventions within the group setting can provide a child with the sense of power and control that comes from solving problems and mastering new experiences, ideas, and skills. As a result, it can help build feelings of confidence and accomplishment. Utilizing play therapy approaches in a group setting maximizes the healing process and therapeutic powers of play (Schaefer & Drewes, 2010).

Group play therapy offers several children at once the ability to utilize the necessary time, space, and treatment approach to heal presenting problems and make therapeutic change across various and multi-dimensional psychological disorders. It is an efficient and time effective way to reach more children at one time (Sweeney et al., 2014). In addition, children benefit from the group dynamics, enhancing peer relationships, problem solving skills, role play, and modeling, and normalization of experiences and symptoms. Children not only benefit from the support of peers, but also have the presence of a therapist who can help them feel heard, understood, and accepted through the healing powers of play (Schaefer & Drewes, 2010). Moreover, group social and play skills training groups and programs have gained popularity, largely because they are developmentally sensitive; developed from solid philosophic and theoretical underpinnings with empirically and evidence-based research showing their positive impact (Bratton et. al., 2005; Reddy et al., 2005).

Not all clinicians are trained or adept in working in a group therapy approach, and especially in bringing in play-based techniques and approaches to use with groups. It requires that the clinician have the tools necessary to use in their therapeutic work. Clinicians need play-based techniques and approaches that are engaging, especially to overcome resistance to the treatment process. The challenge for the group therapist is to provide an atmosphere that is playful, yet offers enough structure. Providing the proper group constellation will allow healing to begin. There are few books available to the play therapist on group play therapy that can guide both the novice and seasoned clinician.

Implementing Play Therapy in Groups: Contemporary Issues in Practice edited jointly by Mellenthin, Stone, and Grant, has come on the scene just in time to meet the demands of dealing with the unique problems in the world. It is a new and innovative edited book that addresses issues such as military families, crisis intervention, sexual abuse, children of divorce, post-adoption, and utilizing body work in treating trauma to name just a few across a wide range of clinical settings.

The editors have succeeded in their aim. They have brought together experienced play therapists from across the globe to share their knowledge, experience, and theoretical perspective in providing the most appropriate group treatment approach depending on the clinical setting they practice in or their particular expertise in clinical areas. The book is meant for not only students new to play therapy, but also professionals who have been working in the field who are interested in exploring different perspectives and experiences of facilitating group play therapy. The editors have given the time and thoughtfulness to highlight special considerations in dealing with specific settings where group play therapy is being implemented, such as tele-mental health, in schools, hospitals, clinics, and residential treatment centers.

Introduction to Groupwork in Play Therapy, by Mellenthin and Willard, opens the book and sets the groundwork and solid foundation for the novice and experienced therapist to start using group play therapy. It briefly discusses the history of group play therapy, the different types of group therapy treatment that is developmentally appropriate for use with children and teens, and introduces the reader to the many ways group work can be utilized in play therapy.

The book then is divided into three parts. Part I covers specific types of contemporary play therapy used in group therapy practice models. There are seven chapters, addressing group work using LEGO® Play by Peabody; Sand Therapy by Armstrong, Foster, and Hickman; Social Skills by Ansari; AutPlay® groups with autistic children by Turner-Bumberry and Grant; Digital Play Therapy by Stone and Ehrig; TraumaPlay® by Goodyear-Brown, Worley, and Rubens; and using groups in telehealth by Fyfe. Part II, with four chapters, focuses on a wide array of specific clinical settings that most clinicians work in where group therapy can be used. Schoonover and Perryman address schools, while Turner and Boles focus on medical/hospital play groups, and Crenshaw and Garrett focuses on residential treatment centers. Mellenthin addresses outpatient mental health settings. Part III, with seven chapters, addresses special populations. Stewart and Echterling address working with military families, Shelby highlights group therapy for victims of natural disasters, and Green and Herdzik focus on children of divorce through a Jungian perspective. Kenney-Noziska addresses group play therapy with sexually abused children, Fraser focuses on unique challenges with children who are adopted out of foster care, Hamilton and Moran discuss groups with neurodiverse children, and a final chapter is devoted to supervision groups by Taylor.

Implementing Play Therapy in Groups: Contemporary Issues in Practice is innovative. This excellent book offers the frontline clinician practical, modern information to implement across challenging settings, diagnoses, and practice environments. The chapters are consistent across the volume in bringing alive the approaches and techniques presented, making it easily applicable for the reader. Chapter authors nicely break down the format of each group therapy session, so the beginner can follow the structure needed to create their own group. Practical case studies and clinical case examples flesh out how each group evolves over time, and offers us insight into the children's journey to finding hope, confidence, and success in their abilities and social interactions.

This gem of a book is indeed a complete compendium, comprehensively detailed for working in group therapy. Readers will be delighted by the style and the substance of the book, by its clarity of language and wealth of specific detail. Much of the subject matter included herein has never been covered before, given the dearth of publications and emphasis on group play therapy. So dear clinician, you can feel confident and be ready to immediately implement group therapy work into your practice. So, get comfortable, dig in, and enjoy reading!

References

Bratton, S., Ray, D., Rhine, T., & Jones, L. (2005). The efficacy of play therapy with children: A meta-analytic review of treatment outcomes. *Professional Psychology: Research and Practice*, 36(4), 376–390.

Ginott, H. (1961). *Group psychotherapy with children: The theory and practice of play therapy*. McGraw Hill.

Reddy, L. A., Files-Hall, T. M., & Schaefer, C. E. (2005). *Empirically based play interventions for children*. American Psychological Association.

Schaefer, C. E. & Drewes, A. A. (2010). *The therapeutic powers of play: 20 core agents of change*. Wiley.

Sweeney, D. & Homeyer, L. (1999). *The handbook of group play therapy*. Jossey-Bass.

Sweeney, D., Baggerly, J., & Ray, D. (2014). *Group play therapy: A dynamic approach*. Routledge.

Introduction and Foundation of Group Play Therapy

Clair Mellenthin and Holly Willard

Group play therapy combines the healing powers of play and the benefits of the group process. The interactive group experience provides connection with other children in the safe and growth-promoting setting of play therapy. Group play therapy can be a powerful intervention, especially when children are experiencing interpersonal and intrapersonal difficulties (Sweeney & Homeyer, 1999). They learn new ways of *being* as they share in the group experience with their peers; they are permitted to communicate in play and learn from one another. Because play is the natural mode of communication in children, they may have increased motivation to play and be expressive around other children (Kottman, 2003). Sweeney (2011) writes, "Group play therapy is the recognition of children's medium of communication (play), combined with the natural benefit of human connection with other children, under the facilitation of trained and caring adult" (p. 227). In the play therapy group, children learn to be more aware of each other and themselves. They will be more in tune with their needs, feelings, and thoughts; and how to appropriately interact with others (Ray, 2011).

In this chapter, we will review the history of group play therapy, the developmental stages of group process, different models of group play therapy, and why the group play therapy process can be so effective in treating a wide range of psychosocial difficulties in children and adolescents.

History of Group Play Therapy

Group therapy was developed in the early 19th century. Over the last century, it has become a central aspect of psychotherapy, well known for its efficacy and utilization across the spectrum of human development. In the late 1800's and early 1900's group work was established as a means to treat and/or educate many adults at one time, which tended to consist of immigrants, poor, or mentally ill (Erford, 2010). Joseph Pratt, a Boston physician is the first known professional to use groups and understand the therapeutic value that group experiences can facilitate. In his treatment with patients who were hospitalized with tuberculosis, he found that the

DOI: 10.4324/9781003094531-101

members began building relationships and caring for one another through the group experience, which, in turn, led to the majority of his patients recovering from ailments which were previously believed to be terminal illnesses (Erford, 2010).

Alfred Adler began conducting groups in the 1920's with children and family members, examining his belief that children's problems and family experiences are interconnected and related. He began a new, systemic format of engaging groups of family members in the therapeutic process and allowing for all voices to be heard – even the very youngest members of the household. This approach became to be known as collective counseling (Erford, 2010). During this same timeframe, Sigmund Freud published the book *Group Psychology and the Analysis of the Ego* (1921), bringing group therapy to the field of psychoanalysis. Jacob Moreno coined the term group psychotherapy in 1932 and the first well-known adult support groups such as Alcoholics Anonymous and formal psychotherapy groups began (Erford, 2010; Paquin, 2021).

It is during this same timeframe that play therapy was born out of the field of psychoanalysis. In the early Child Guidance Clinics in the UK and Europe, child psychoanalysts treated and formally observed groups of children playing and interacting together. In the 1950's, group play therapy began to be established in the United States in the Child Guidance Clinics and became to be recognized for its efficacy and ability to promote change in behaviors, decreased emotional distress, and improved social skills (Ginott, 1958). These early American play therapists utilized Virginia Axline's model of child centered play therapy in their group work and found that through the group experience, the therapeutic relationship was enhanced, as was the social and emotional relationships between the child clients (1958). Ginott published several articles in the 1950's and 1960's regarding his work with children in play therapy and wrote the first book on a group play therapy practice model in his 1961 classic book *Group Psychotherapy with Children*. Over thirty years would pass until another group play therapy book would be published, *The Handbook of Group Play Therapy* (Sweeney & Homeyer, 1999), although the field of play therapy was far from stagnant during these ensuing decades. Another two decades would pass until the next book *Group Play Therapy: A Dynamic Approach* (Sweeney et al., 2014) was published.

Throughout the last decade, group play therapy has been widely researched. Several research studies have looked at the efficacy of using various treatment models. The review of studies on group play therapy by Meany-Walen, Bullis, Kottman, and Taylor (2015) showed positive results for improving children's functioning in several settings and a variety of therapeutic goals. In group play therapy with pre-school aged children, it was shown to correlate to positive results for improving children's social interactions, self-awareness, and self-regulation (Chinekesh et al., 2014; Stone & Stark, 2013). Child-centered group play therapy was found to be effective in improving kindergarten students' social skill development (Kascsak, 2013). In the research related to the effects of group play therapy in school age children, Woolf (2011) showed participation in group play therapy led to improvement students' self-esteem, ability to interact responsibility, and emotional well-being.

Research on group play therapy with traumatized children has also found empirical support. Meany-Walen et al. (2015) referenced research showing group play therapy being beneficial for children exposed to domestic violence (Thompson & Trice-Black, 2012), abuse and/or other traumatic events (Gil, 2006; Homeyer, 1999), death and loss (Le Vieux, 1999), and hospitalization (Lingnell & Dunn, 1999). Gil and Drewes' (2005) multicultural research found that group play therapy is effective for children from various cultures, gender, and ethnicities. This is important research, as it gives empirical evidence on the nature of group play therapy to treat a wide range of emotional and psychosocial difficulties in children.

Group Play Therapy in Practice

Hobbs (1951) wrote,

> It is one thing to be understood and accepted by a therapist, it is considerably a more potent experience to be understood and accepted by several people who are also honestly sharing their feelings in a joint search for a more satisfying way of life.
>
> (p. 281)

The yearning to be seen and known is a crucial tenet of attachment theory and human relationships. Group play therapy is "the natural union of two effective therapeutic modalities" with similar core values and desired outcomes (Sweeney & Homeyer, 1999, p. 3). Both group therapy and play therapy are evidence-based models of treatment, centered on a dynamic process of relationship-building, and are committed to a creative and dynamic therapeutic process (1999).

In discussing the power of group play therapy, Landreth (1999) postulated:

> In this relationship, children learn from each other, encourage each other, support each other, work out difficulties, share in pain and joy, discover what it is like to help each other, and discover that they are capable of giving as well as receiving help. In this unique relationship children discover their uniqueness as well as their similarities.
>
> (p. xi)

Most importantly, the child discovers that they are not alone. It is through the group experience, that a child learns they are not the only ones who may be experiencing a challenging home environment, loneliness, grief, or mental illness. It is by finding and experiencing acceptance that a child learns that they are loved and loveable, worthy of connection and friendship.

Benefits of Group Play Therapy

The advantages and implications of group play therapy are numerous and diverse. Group play therapy gives the child an opportunity to explore their strengths and challenges in the presence of other children who will provide feedback, acceptance, and support (Ray, 2011). Since the early writings of Ginott, researchers and practitioners have observed that children are much more comfortable in engaging in play therapy when other children are present (Ginott, 1961). They experience vicarious and induced catharsis through their shared play (Ray, 2011). Indirect and direct teaching and learning takes place as the child learns new coping skills, the courage to explore emotional and behavioral expressions, and increase problem-solving skills (Drewes & Schafer, 2014; Sweeney & Homeyer, 1999). Children also can engage in reality testing and limit setting, as they are able to experiment with new behaviors within a safe environment (Sweeney & Homeyer, 1999). Lastly, a child is able to engage in positive interactions with a caring, trusted adult and other same-age children, which is all too often lacking in their life experiences.

The developments in the field of neurobiology show additional benefits of play therapy and the impact of group play therapy on a neurological level (Kestly, 2014). Humans are hardwired to establish social connections with others and group play therapy provides an opportunity for children to not only connect with the therapist, but connect with other children. With the discovery of mirror neurons, brain cells that fire in reaction to perceiving another's actions as if one performed the action itself, the vital role of playing *together* is increased. There is a powerful neurological process that occurs while viewing other group member's play, which can be literally transformative (Schermer, 2010).

Practicalities of Group Play Therapy

Size of Group

Depending on the theoretical orientation of the play therapist, as well as the type of group, the size of the group may differ significantly. The age of group members may also influence the group size, as generally therapists hold smaller groups for younger children and larger groups for teens. Younger children need more structure and therapeutic support and are typically not as comfortable in the large group experience. For example, it is recommended that Child-Centered Play Therapy groups consist of 2–3 members to allow for the child to have enough room to move freely and for the therapist to be attuned to the child's needs and multiple dynamics taking place (Ray, 2011). Other group modalities can offer more structured activities, lending to larger group size.

Gender Composition

Depending on the age of the child group participants, the gender composition changes in the group format. For young children, gender is not as important or social awareness of gender norms have not been developed. However, as children become older, they become more entrenched in gender patterns and focus on differences in play and verbalization. Due to these developmental differences after the age of six, some models recommended that same gendered groups of children occur (Ray, 2011). In contemporary times, as the concept of gender has become much more fluid, more research and awareness are needed on the importance of acceptance and the impact of gender segregation that takes place in the latency age of development.

Age

Younger children historically establish their relationships with each other in a hierarchical manner, using age as the primary decisive factor in leadership. One well-known guideline, especially with Child-Centered Play Therapy groups, is to match children within one-year chronological age to avoid inequality that accompanies age differences (Ray, 2011). Another way to divide children by age is by school setting. For example, the child's grade in primary school, secondary school, and high school would determine their placement within a group. More importantly, the age differences in the group should not put any members in an at-risk situation, such as a minor teenager in a group with young adults.

Cultural Competency

Multicultural competency refers to the clinician's awareness, knowledge, and skills to engage in a course of actions that maximizes the optimal development of the client and their immediate systems (Sue & Torino, 2005). Being mindful and cognizant of the intersectionality of culture, race, ethnicity, sexuality, neurodiversity, religion, socioeconomic status, gender, etc. is important in creating a cohesive group experience for both the child participants as well as the treatment provider. Culture is a shared human experience that encompasses shared values, history, and customs that frequently result in a shared group identity (Chen et al., 2008). It is the therapist's responsibility to pursue multi-cultural competence through education, training, consultation, and supervision to acquire knowledge and skills in providing services for a culturally diverse clientele. Creating culturally safe spaces is a critical aspect of play therapy that at times in overlooked and undervalued.

Group Composition Considerations

When composing groups, the play therapist also needs to consider the personality, behavior, and characteristics of each group member. Therapists should consider if the group members will support each other's process in the group or if some group members will shut down other group members' ability to participate (i.e., overwhelm, distract, or intimidate). The biggest consideration is to make sure that each individual client will feel physically and emotionally safe in the group. A facilitator should aim to obtain some balance in groups in personality and gender identity. For example, if two withdrawn children are in the group, then it may be helpful to balance with two outgoing or assertive children (Ray, 2011).

Open-Ended or Closed-Ended Group

An open-ended group means that the group is ongoing and group members can be added to the group at any time. A closed-ended group usually has a predetermined number of sessions and group membership remains intact for the duration of the group. Whether a group is open- or closed-ended depends on many factors including: therapeutic model, group setting, purpose of the group, and needs of clientele.

Length of Group Session

Therapists should consider the attention span of the children in group when determining the length of the group session. Generally, the younger the child, the shorter the group session. As a rough guideline, play therapists should consider the following developmentally appropriate recommendations: preschool children's groups should be 30–45 minutes, elementary age children 45–60 minutes, and for teenagers, groups can be up to 90 minutes. With older children and adolescents, an activity or intervention in group of some kind is recommended to elicit play and creativity.

Group Set Up

A playroom set up specifically for groups is the ideal setting for running play therapy groups. However, an adequately sized room (at least twelve by fifteen feet) with steady furniture is suggested (Sweeney & Homeyer, 1999). Materials for group play therapy should include a variety of materials that facilitate a wide range of creative and emotional expression, facilitate exploratory play, engage children's interests, and allow for unstructured play (Sweeney et al., 2014).

Categories of Play Therapy Groups

There are two main types of group work that are practiced by mental health clinicians. **Treatment groups** focus on helping individuals achieve emotional and mental health and wellness through the development of social skills, education, and therapy (Hepworth et al., 2017). Members of a treatment group often are involved in a dynamic relationship, where interactions between members occurs as communication is open and engaging. In **Task groups**, the focus may be on the "group as a whole", meaning that the change mechanism occurs within the system as the group works together to achieve an end goal (Hepworth et al., 2017).

Within the treatment group paradigm, play therapists may find themselves facilitating different types of group work with their clients. Each type of group serves a specific treatment purpose and clinicians should be mindful of the treatment objectives, developmental stages of clients, and clinical appropriateness in engaging in group work. Toseland and Rivas (2009) refined their classification of treatment groups that are characterized by their clinical purpose:

1 Support Groups: Help group members cope with life stressors through the use of social support and enhancing coping skills. This may or may not be facilitated by a mental health clinician.
2 Educational Groups: Help group members learn about themselves and their world. Psychoeducation groups are common in teaching social and relationship skills.
3 Growth Groups: Help members to improve self-awareness, personal growth, and self-improvement. This type of group differs from other groups in that the focus is on promoting socioemotional health rather than alleviating symptoms.
4 Therapy Groups: Help members learn new behaviors, coping strategies, or rehabilitate themselves following a traumatic experience. The primary focus is on remediation and rehabilitation (Hepworth et al., 2017).
5 Socialization Groups: Help group members work through transitions through developmental stages, environments, or role changes. Members are taught positive interpersonal relationships and/or social skills.

Stages of Group Development

For the purposes of this chapter, the Tuckman (1965) model of small group development will be discussed. Although there are other models of group therapy, this model has withstood the test of time and continues to be popular, in terms of research, academia, and practice (Bonebright, 2010). Tuckman's four-stage model consists of forming, storming, norming, and preforming stages. This model occurs throughout various treatment models and is important to understand when facilitating group play therapy.

Forming

The forming stage begins as group members are introduced to one another and rapport and relationships begin to bloom. In this initial stage, group members become oriented to the task, develop group rules, and test boundaries in relationships and behavior (Bonebright, 2010).

Storming

The second stage of this group developmental model is the storming phase. This stage represents a stage of group conflict. In this stage of development, there is often a lack of relational cohesion between group members, with Tuckman stating, "group members become hostile toward one another and toward a therapist or trainer as a means of expressing their individuality and resisting the formation of group structure" (1965, p. 386). Each group member is attempting to develop and define their role in the group membership.

Norming

The third stage is Norming. In this stage, the group begins to accept one another, with all their quirks and idiosyncrasies. Roles and norms are accepted and the group develops much more cohesion in working towards their treatment goals and objectives (Bonebright, 2010). Tuckman (1965) stated that in this stage, the group becomes an entity as members develop in-group feeling and seek to maintain and perpetuate the group.

Performing

This final stage of performing occurs as the group develops "functional role relatedness" (Tuckman, 1965) or in layman's terms, the group members are able to work together as their authentic selves. The roles and responsibilities within the group shift and change, as the group is able to problem-solve, practice, and incorporate new knowledge into their functioning and relationships.

Ethical and Legal Considerations

Due to the complexity of facilitating play therapy groups, therapists need to have proper training and supervised experience in the field. Therapists should have training in play therapy, the group process, specific therapeutic models, and the therapeutic issue being treated. Even experienced play therapists need consultation and support from other play therapists (Ray, 2011; Sweeney & Homeyer, 1999). Countertransference in group can be magnified, especially when there is not cohesion between group members and the facilitator. Facilitators can feel frustrated or overwhelmed with the chaos of the group process, as well as feel helpless to elicit change in the early stages of group development. Co-facilitating the group with another play therapist can be immensely helpful, especially if the number of group participants is larger than four children.

Therapists need to be aware of and follow ethical and legal guidelines of their corresponding professional organizations. The Association of Play Therapy Best Practices on Group Work (2020) recommends:

- Screening: The play therapist selects clients for group play therapy whose needs are compatible and conducive to the therapeutic process and well-being of each client.
- Protecting Clients: Play therapists using group play therapy take reasonable precautions in protecting clients from physical and psychological trauma.
- Confidentiality in Groups: Play therapists explain to group members, and/or their legal guardians (when the group includes those who are legally under guardianship) the importance of maintaining confidentiality outside of the group, instruct them in methods for doing so and make special efforts to ensure confidentiality in settings where it may be more readily compromised, such as schools or inpatient/residential treatment settings. Rules for the group and consequence of breaking the rules should be clear to all group members. If a member of the group cannot abide by the rules of the group, consequences need to be enforced for the protection of others (Association of Play Therapy Best Practices, A9: Group Work).

Informed consent or parental permission must be obtained prior to participation. As part of the informed consent, the purpose of the group needs to be identified. Children and guardians should be informed of confidentiality limits. Children should have the opportunity to participate or leave the group (Ray, 2011; Sweeney & Homeyer, 1999).

Conclusion

During the current experience of a global pandemic, where connections through social relationships are being challenged in a degree that has never been seen, the need for people to interact in therapeutic groups is unsurmountable (Inchausti et al., 2020). With the advances in telehealth, group play therapy can be provided online to minimize health concerns, increase social and emotional connection to others, as well as provide a platform for support, psychoeducation, and empowerment. It can also be facilitated in a safe, socially distanced manner to provide contact and experience. Group play therapy is a powerful intervention for children, teens, and adults. Group play therapy presents opportunities for the individual child to explore themselves in the context of a social environment and have other children provide feedback, acceptance, and support. Group play therapy has been utilized throughout the last several decades, however, there continues to be a need for further research and application. The specifics of each group should be considered based on therapeutic model, setting, client needs, and resources available.

References

Association for Play Therapy. (2020). Best Practices A9: Group Work. *APT.* https://cdn.ymaws.com/www.a4pt.org/resource/resmgr/publications/apt_best_practices_-_june_20.pdf.

Bonebright, D. (2010). 40 years of storming: A historical review of Tuckman's model of small group development. *Human Resource Development International,* 13(1), 111–120.

Chen, E. C., Kakadu, D., & Bolzano, J. (2008). Multicultural competence and evidence-based practice in group therapy. *Journal of Clinical Psychology,* 64(11), 1261–1278.

Chinekesh, A., Kamalian, M., Eltemasi, M., Chinekesh, S., & Alavi, M. (2014). The effect of group play therapy on social-emotional skills in pre-school children. *Global Journal of Health Science,* 6, 163–167.

Drewes, A. A. & Schaefer, C. E. (Eds.) (2014). *The therapeutic powers of play.* (2nd ed.). Wiley.

Erford, B. T. (2010). *Group work in the schools.* Prentice Hall.

Gil, E. (2006). *Helping abused and traumatized children: Integrating directive and nondirective approaches.* Guilford Press.

Gil, E. & Drewes, A. A. (Eds.) (2005). *Cultural issues in play therapy.* Guilford Press.

Ginott, H. G. (1958). Play group therapy: A theoretical framework. *International Journal of Group Psychotherapy,* 8(1), 410.

Ginott, H. (1961). *Group psychotherapy with children: The theory and practice of play therapy.* McGraw-Hill.

Hepworth, D. H., Rooney, R. H., Rooney, G. D., & Strom-Gottfried, K. (2017). *Direct social work practice: Theory and skills.* Cengage Learning.

Hobbs, N. (1951). Group-centered therapy. In C. R. Rogers (Ed.), *Client-centered therapy.* (pp. 278–319). Houghton Mifflin.

Homeyer, L. E. (1999). Group play therapy with sexually abused children. In D. S. Sweeney, & L. E. Homeyer (Eds.), *The handbook of group play therapy* (pp. 299–318). Jossey-Bass.

Inchausti, F., MacBeth, A., Hasson-Ohayon, I., & Dimaggio, G. (2020). Psychological Intervention and COVID-19: What we know so far and what we can do. *Journal of Contemporary Psychotherapy,* 1–8. Advance online publication.

Kascsak, T. M. (2013). The impact of child-centered group play therapy on social skills development of kindergarten children. *Dissertation Abstracts International: Section A. Humanities and Social Sciences,* 73, 2013.

Kestly, T. A. (2014). *The interpersonal neurobiology of play: Brain-building interventions for emotional well-being.* W. W. Norton & Co.

Kottman, T. (2003). *Partners in play* (2nd ed.). American Counseling Association.

Landreth, G. L. (1999). Foreword. In D. S. Sweeney & L. E. Homeyer (Eds.), *The handbook of group play therapy: How to do it, how it works, whom it's best for.* (pp. xi–xii). Jossey-Bass.

Le Vieux, J. (1999). Group play therapy with grieving children. In D. S. Sweeney & L. E. Homeyer (Eds.), *The handbook of group play therapy* (pp. 375–388). Jossey-Bass.

Lingnell, L. & Dunn, L. (1999). Group play: Wholeness and healing for the hospitalized child. In D. S. Sweeney & L. E. Homeyer (Eds.), *The handbook of group play therapy* (pp. 359–374). Jossey-Bass.

Meany-Walen, K. K., Bullis, Q., Kottman, T., & Taylor, D. D. (2015). Group Adlerian play therapy with children with off-task behaviors. *The Journal for Specialists in Group Work*, 40(3), 294–314.

Paquin, A. (2021). A brief history of group therapy as a field and the representation of women in its development. *International Journal of Group Psychotherapy*, 71(1), 13–80.

Ray, D. C. (2011). *Advanced play therapy: Essential conditions, knowledge, and skills for child practice.* Routledge.

Schermer V. L. (2010). Mirror neurons: Their implications for group psychotherapy. *International Journal of Group Psychotherapy*, 60, 487–513.

Stone, S. & Stark, M. (2013). Structured play therapy groups for preschoolers: Facilitating the emergence of social competence. *International Journal of Group Psychotherapy*, 63(1), 25–50.

Sue, D. S. & Torino, G. C. (2005). Racial-cultural competence: Awareness, knowledge, and skills. In R. T. Carter (Ed.), *Handbook of racial-cultural psychology and counseling: Training and practice, Vol. 2* (pp. 3–18). Wiley.

Sweeney, D. S. (2011). Group play therapy. In C. E. Schaefer (Ed.), *Foundations of play therapy* (2nd ed.) (pp. 227–252). Wiley.

Sweeney, D. S. & Homeyer, L. E. (Eds.) (1999). *The handbook of group play therapy: How to do it, how it works, whom it's best for.* Jossey-Bass.

Sweeney, D. S., Baggerly, J. N., & Ray, D. C. (2014). *Group play therapy: A dynamic approach.* Routledge.

Thompson, E. & Trice-Black, S. (2012). School-based group interventions for children exposed to domestic violence. *Journal of Family Violence*, 27, 233–241.

Toseland, R. W. & Rivas, R. F. (2009). *An introduction to group work practice* (6th ed.). Allyn & Bacon.

Tuckman, B. W. (1965). Developmental sequence in small groups. *Psychological Bulletin*, 65(6), 384–399.

Woolf, A. (2011). Everyone playing in class: A group play provision for enhancing the emotional well-being of children in school. *British Journal of Special Education*, 38, 178–190.

Part I

Group Play Therapy Practice Models

1 Constructing Together

Therapeutic Applications of LEGO® Serious Play®

Mary Anne Peabody

LEGO® bricks are among the world's most iconic play objects. These small objects form a "system of play" designed on the principle that all bricks interlock and interrelate (Gauntlett, 2015). As such, newly manufactured bricks still connect with the original 1958 bricks and bricks from one kit are easily integrated with other kits (Gauntlett, 2015). This ingenious system of play contributes to why LEGO® play is universally cherished by both children and adults (Robertson & Breen, 2013). This concept of universality across the life span also makes LEGO® play an ideal choice for group work experiences that utilize object-mediated communication. Object-mediated communication uses tangible objects to invite shared dialogue (McGuire et al., 2015). When the objects used are LEGO® bricks, the bricks become the focal point for inquiry and the representation of thoughts and feelings to promote deeper understanding.

One specific group approach that uses LEGO® bricks as objects for communication is LEGO® SERIOUS PLAY® (LSP). LSP is a facilitated methodology that utilizes the creative power of LEGO® bricks to generate a psychologically safe environment for problem solving through storytelling (Kristiansen & Rasmussen, 2014). The method involves a structured progression of activities based on (a) creating a model; (b) attributing metaphorical meaning to the model; and (c) sharing the meaning with the others in the group.

While originally developed to address complex problem-solving needs in the business sector (Kristiansen & Rasmussen, 2014) there is a growing interest by mental health professionals in adapting the traditional model of LSP to therapeutic group venues (Harn, 2018; Kestly, 2014; Peabody, 2015). Accordingly, when the facilitator is a licensed clinical mental health professional with specialized training in group work and the LSP methodology, a powerful multiplying effect can occur (Peabody & Noyes, 2017). To this end, it is not the bricks but rather the skilled facilitation of the process that produces change.

Capitalizing on the appeal of LEGO® play across the life span, this chapter begins with an overview of several current therapeutic applications, followed by the theoretical underpinnings of the specific LSP methodology.

DOI: 10.4324/9781003094531-1

Next, research on both the traditional LSP approach and adaptations into therapeutic applications are discussed with an invitation for continual exploration and research into the use of LSP into therapeutic venues. Then, a case example is presented that utilizes an adult group play therapy model to illustrate the integration of the therapeutic factors of group work (Yalom, 1995) with the LSP methodology (Kristiansen & Rasmussen, 2014) conceptualized through a resiliency model (Umhoefer et al., 2015).

Overview of LEGO® Play in Therapeutic Contexts

Only recently has the use of LEGO® bricks within therapeutic contexts appeared in literature (Harn, 2017; Legoff et al., 2014; Peabody, 2015). Play therapist, Theresa Kestly (2014) wrote about LSP in family therapy, Babs and Boniwell (2016) situated the traditional LSP model into a positive psychology framework, and this author adapted LSP principles within play therapy clinical supervision (Peabody, 2015). Psychologist, Pay-Ling Harn (2018) explored a LEGO® facilitative method in clinical practice with a focus on social connection, emotion conversion, cognitive development, and action taking. Harn (2017) also used a strength-centered LSP workshop model with survivors of domestic violence and a group model with clients experiencing stress (Harn & Hsiao, 2018).

Specific to children, Thomsen (2018) explored the therapeutic use of LEGO® bricks for boosting children's emotional well-being in her book entitled, *Therabuild* and Tulluck (2020) published *Brick-Based Counseling*, a practitioner-friendly book to support children's social-emotional learning. Currently, the LEGO® Education company has several products designed by teachers and educational specialists that utilize story building across traditional academic subjects, and early intervention products that promote feeling recognition and expression.

Finally, the two approaches most frequently found in the literature are LEGO®-based therapy and LSP. The two approaches are markedly different in terms of their targeted audience, learning objectives, facilitation processes, and overt activities. Next, we explore these disparate approaches in greater detail.

LEGO®-based Therapy

LEGO®-based therapy (LBT) is a well-researched directive group social skills intervention for school-age children with autism, social communication needs, dysregulation issues, and other neurodevelopmental disorders that is typically offered in education or after-school settings (Legoff et al., 2014; MacCormack et al., 2015). LBT capitalizes on LEGO® bricks as a predictable, systematic, multilevel construction toy that provides intrinsically structured tasks that many children with autism are both attracted to and motivated by through active engagement (Baron-Cohen, 2008; Owens, et al., 2008).

In small groups, children are assigned designated roles, such as engineer, supplier, and builder. Within these roles, children strive to communicate and follow social rules to complete specific LEGO® builds. Each activity requires verbal and non-verbal communication, the development of social communication skills such as sharing, following social rules, making eye contact, and joint problem-solving. Numerous studies and books have been conducted and published on this approach, so readers are encouraged to explore the literature surrounding this intervention in more depth (Legoff et al., 2014; MacCormack et al., 2015).

LEGO® Serious Play® (LSP)

LSP is a facilitated communication methodology that aims to help groups solve a problem, reach a common goal, foster insight and self-awareness (LEGO® Serious Play, 2010). LSP seeks to create group experiences that unlock participant potential through breaking habitual thinking, unearthing new insights, and creating deep meaning making (Kristiansen & Rasmussen, 2014). Unlike some therapeutic group experiences, the LSP expectation is that all participants will "lean in and participate" so that everyone builds, everyone shares, and everyone speaks (James, 2015).

Therefore, the process of using brick objects to express ideas metaphorically is carefully paced and modeled by the facilitator to create a psychologically safe environment for inclusive group sharing. As group participants share their experiences and reflect on their feelings to make meaning, both emotional expression and group cohesion is accelerated (Peabody & Noyes, 2017). Consequentially, there is growing interest by mental health professionals to become certified in the LSP full methodology to deeply understand, successfully facilitate, and intentionally adapt this approach with therapeutic populations (Peabody, 2015; Sutton, 2012).

The professional training involved to learn the traditional LSP methodology includes several facilitated steps and seven applications that become increasingly more complex over time (Kristiansen & Rasmussen, 2014). Depending on the goals, objectives, purpose, and time constraints, an LSP group may progress through all seven application stages, or only focus on the first few applications. The bricks used within LSP are specialized LEGO® kits that supply a mix of metaphoric pieces and general LEGO® bricks to invite symbolic 3-dimensional modeling that aids in story creation.

Theories Supporting LSP Group Work

Knitted together from psychology, behavioral sciences, education, and neuroscience, the theoretical underpinnings supporting LSP can be considered an amalgamation of interdisciplinary fields. Together these junctures present a coherent understanding of how people learn and how group dynamics influence this learning. The melding of psychological and behavioral science principles with educational practices is not new, and this next section high-lights prominent areas of convergence among the LSP theories most applic-able to therapeutic play therapy groups.

Constructivism

LSP is grounded in the theory of constructivism, developed by Jean Piaget (1964) who considered humans to be active theory builders rather than passive absorbers of information with the ability to construct, rearrange, and deconstruct knowledge-based experiences. In constructivist theory, the process of meaning-making and constructing knowledge is understood to have both individual and social components, so that individuals not only learn from their own thinking processes, but also by accessing and inter-secting with the learning of others (McAuliffe & Eriksen, 2011).

Constructionism

A colleague of Piaget's (1964), Seymour Papert (1999) extended the con-structivism theory to what he called constructionism theory. Papert's theory asserted learning was further deepened when people engaged in constructing something external to themselves (Kristiansen & Rasmussen, 2014; Papert & Harel, 1991). Papert (1999) believed that the hand-mind process of "thinking through your fingers," engaged various modes of thought, creative energies, and imagination. According to Papert & Harel (1991) this hand-mind experience allowed abstract ideas to become visual and tangible, resulting in deeper understanding and discoveries of thought that otherwise might not be accessible.

Neuroscience Principles

The contributions of neuroscientific principles to mental health treatment have provided therapists with a knowledge base and vocabulary helpful when explaining play therapy to adults. Due to a societal association of play being linked to childhood or considered something frivolous, engaging adults in play-based interventions takes intentional planning, pacing, and language (Badenoch & Kestly, 2015; Walsh, 2019). Some adults may give more cred-ibility to a scientifically grounded explanation of why and how play inter-ventions are helpful. Kestly (2014) encourages play therapists to understand the neurobiology of a storytelling brain at play when explaining why play, and specifically LSP, is the intervention of choice to meet treatment goals.

Research Supporting LSP

There is a burgeoning research base covering traditional LSP methodology with studies exploring the impact on strategic innovation and thinking

(Statler et al., 2011), leadership development (Dykes, 2018; Holliday et al., 2007; Peabody & Turesky, 2018) and within higher education coursework (Dann, 2018; Nerantzi & James, 2019). Research studies within higher education have examined: accelerated group cohesion (Peabody & Noyes, 2017), group members sense of identity (Gauntlett, 2007), creative confidence (Dykes, 2018) and adult student learning engagement (Chung, 2019). In contrast, there is a paucity of studies exploring LSP therapeutically except for those previously mentioned by Harn and colleagues (Harn, 2017; Harn & Hsiao, 2018), thereby illuminating a gap in the literature and offering new frontiers for exploration.

Adult Group Work

Prolific play therapy author Charles Schaefer (2003) and other mental health professionals have endorsed the value of play with adults (Brown & Vaughan, 2010; Grant et al., 2021; Gray 2009). While many play therapists specialize in working with children, play is equally important for the well-being of adults as the play circuitry of humans remains central at all ages (Badenoch & Kestly, 2015). Badenoch and Kestly (2015) stated play therapists can be the wise voice, at the right moments with adults, to make a linkage between play and inner self-awareness (p. 536). Similarly, psychiatrist Lenore Terr (1999) stated that play is the key to unlocking the door to ourselves regardless of age (p. 40).

Just as play has specific therapeutic powers that elicit change (Schaefer & Drewes, 2014), so does clinical group work. Yalom (1995) presented several therapeutic group work factors as mechanisms of change and while a detailed exploration of all the factors is beyond the scope of this chapter, readers are encouraged to explore his work to guide clinical decision making. In the following case example, we examine three of Yalom's (Yalom & Leszcz, 2005) therapeutic factors of group work including: group cohesiveness and belonging; the concept of universality where what seems unique is often a similar or identical experience of another group member or a "we are all in the same boat" phenomenon; and altruism which is both giving and receiving support. These selected factors help members gain insight into themselves and their relationships with others.

Case Example

This case is a composite of group experiences with non-deployed parents of children attending a public elementary school in an active military community. Deployment is considered a type of ambiguous loss as it is embedded in uncertain changes which are difficult to manage (Cohen-Konrad, 2013; Huebner et al., 2007). Deployment-related ambiguous loss often brings on anticipation, worry, fears, and shifts in routines, tasks, and family structure (Huebner et al., 2007). While many non-deployed spouses/partners demonstrate flexibility and resiliency, others struggle with symptoms consistent with depression, anxiety, and sleep difficulties (Mansfield et al., 2010) or may present as physically or emotionally drained (Kees & Rosenblum, 2015).

Boss (2006) suggests that ambiguous loss be treated in family, group, or community-based approaches rather than individual approaches to create social support, a sense of belonging, and the universality factor. As such, the Pathways to Resilience (P2R)-Military Families model was selected as the conceptual framework for the group experiences (Umhoefer et al., 2015). The model is an extension of the original Pathways to Resilience model and includes four factors: reaching out, making meaning, facilitating emotional regulation, and enabling successful coping (Echterling et al., 2005). The P2R-Military Families model adds two more dimensions: addressing the deployment cycle; and acknowledging and addressing the changing roles and responsibilities within the family (Umhoefer et al., 2015).

Parent groups were held in the naturalistic setting of the elementary school to create a shared sense of identity and to build a social support network congruent with the "reaching out" factor of the P2R-Military Families model. The groups utilized a phased process over seven weeks that included an adaptation of the LSP methodology for object mediated communication. Four of the seven LSP applications were introduced: individual models and stories, shared models and stories, creating a landscape, and making connections (Kristiansen & Rasmussen, 2014).

Beginning Phase

The goals in the beginning phase were to familiarize the parents with logistics, group expectations and norms, learning objectives, and specific information about the LSP process. After this initial explanation, the first LSP build was introduced. The purpose of the first build was to allow parents to become familiar with the specialized LSP kit pieces and the sequenced prompt-build-share process. The parents were allowed 3 to 5 minutes to build a brick "creature or animal" from a limited number of bricks and to briefly share what they built with the group. Next each parent was asked to metaphorically explain how their brick creature compared with parenting and military life. This introductory transition into metaphorical sharing is key to the LSP process and liberates participants to tell rich stories with simple builds (Blair & Rillo, 2016; Peabody & Noyes, 2017).

During this phase, the therapist was co-creating a psychological sense of safety through validation of parental stories and encouraging supportive responses amongst group members. Psychological safety includes perceptions of the consequences of taking interpersonal risks, such as contributing ideas in a group context (Edmondson, 1999). A basic LSP principle is that the models and their metaphorical meanings belong to the builder, so there is no right or wrong way to build or to share the associated story. To this end, the process guides group participants to accept the meaning from the builder as that individuals' reality which also contributes to group interactional safety (Kristiansen & Rasmussen, 2014).

Goals for the second week focused on continuing to build psychological safety and group cohesion. The group members were given two directive prompts. Parents were asked to build two models that metaphorically represented the positive and difficult aspects of parenting during deployment. The dialogue quickly cascaded into emotionally rich stories. Positive brick stories were often related to the emotion of pride: including pride of service, in belonging to a military community, in managing "quasi-single parenthood" and in coping under constant uncertainty. Difficult narrative models centered on emotions including: fear and worry for the livelihood of their spouse/partner, occasional resentment of their spouse/partner related to solo parenting, and fatigue or exhaustion due to feeling a need to be positive for their children. Parents shared confusion, shame, and vulnerability-laced stories around the military cultural messaging of "being emotionally strong" throughout the cycle of deployment. The models and story dialogue aligned with several factors in the P2R-Military Families model including: addressing the deployment cycle; emotional regulation around expression of emotions throughout different deployment phases; making meaning of how deployment fits into their sense of self and their families story; and addressing changing roles and responsibilities.

Middle Phase

During the middle phase, the group goals and objectives shifted to successful coping strategies while further establishing trust, relatedness, and sharing. Specific prompts for the brick builds focused on helping parents think of times when deployment was not a problem or when they were able to successfully cope. Additional prompts asked parents to build metaphoric representations of family values, hopes, dreams, and future outcomes.

During this phase, the therapist introduced three new LSP applications: shared building, landscape, and making connections (Kristiansen & Rasmussen, 2014). During the shared build, parents selected one significant part of their individual build to place on the center of the table to co-construct a "mega-story shared build". Different group members took turns sharing their perceived version of the mega-story as they attempted to capture both individual and communal experiences, building experiences of group cohesion and universality.

In the creating a landscape application, the therapist facilitated the group to see similarities, differences, and patterns among the individual models without losing any original meanings (Kristiansen & Rasmussen, 2014).

Next, during the making connections application, the therapist added specialized LEGO® pieces of chains, links, strings, and tubes. Parents made physical connections from their models to other models. The choice of connector material also had symbolic meaning, for example: the difference between using a chain, ladder, string, or flexible tube represented how and why the connection existed (Kristiansen & Rasmussen, 2014). Then a facilitated group reflection step occurred where the therapist invited discussion on connections, insights, surprises, and comments.

End Phase

While acknowledging feelings around ending any therapeutic group experience is important, it is especially true with military families who regularly experience transitions, goodbyes, and relocations. Therefore, in the final phase, group objectives were to integrate and make meaning of the group experience, to extend invitations for social support beyond the group, and to celebrate healthy goodbyes.

The final prompt was to build a model that represented individual learnings from the overall LSP group experience. Themes of validation from others, freedom to play and create laughter with other adults, and permission to break down the facade of "being strong all the time" were re-authored into their final LEGO® builds. The group work factor of altruism was clearly expressed by parents as they shared the positive experience of giving and receiving support (Yalom & Leszcz, 2005). Several parents expressed that by providing support and encouragement to others they felt less isolated, which aligned with the factors inherent in the P2R-Military Families model (Umhoefer et al., 2015). By externally using LEGO® bricks in object-mediated communication, the parents symbolically expressed thoughts, feelings, and mutual support for one another.

Conclusion

LEGO® Serious Play® is a structured facilitation methodology for group work that combines LEGO® model creation and metaphoric storytelling for active engagement. While empirical support for the use of LSP with therapeutic populations is in its nascent stage, the groundwork of evidence is promising. This chapter capitalized on the universal appeal of LEGO® play across the life span (Kristiansen & Rasmussen, 2014) by introducing an integrative multi-model therapeutic group approach for object mediated communication.

LSP leads to individual and collective learning, development, and growth. As LSP requires openness and honesty, it can be a highly sensitive process that requires the facilitator to co-create and monitor a psychologically safe social environment. In doing so, mutual respect and acceptance of differences and individuality can occur. A skilled play therapist can combine the power of group work with play therapy to capitalize on the capacity of the LEGO® system of play to build, deconstruct, re-build, and connect with others. This integrative group work approach offers a structured play-based experience where positive emotional growth and problem solving can be amplified and accelerated (Peabody & Noyes, 2017).

In conclusion, the LEGO® brand name is derived from the Danish words, leg godt, meaning "play well" (LEGO® Foundation, 2018). Extending, this "play well" message into group play therapy encourages competent therapists to embrace an integrative approach with clients to enhance inner awareness and social growth across the life span. Let us continue to provide therapeutic spaces for others to construct together and to "play well".

References

Babs, M. & Boniwell, I. (2016). *LEGO® Serious Play for positive psychology.* http://buildandshare.net/product/book-LEGO®-serious-play-for-positive-psychology/.

Badenoch, B. & Kestly, T. (2015). Exploring the neuroscience of healing play at every age. In D. A. Crenshaw & A. L. Stewart (Eds.), *Play therapy: A comprehensive guide to theory and practice* (pp. 524–538). Guilford.

Baron-Cohen, S. (2008). Autism, hypersystemizing, and truth. *The Quarterly Journal of Experimental Psychology, 61*(1), 64–75.

Blair, S. & Rillo, M. (2016). *Serious work: How to facilitate meetings and workshops using the LEGO® Serious Play.* ProMeet.

Boss, P. (2006). *Loss, trauma, and resilience: Therapeutic work with ambiguous loss.* W. W. Norton & Co.

Brown, S. & Vaughan, C. (2010). *Play: How it shapes the brain, opens the imagination, and invigorates the soul.* Penguin.

Chung, T. K. Y. (2019). *Play to learn: A phenomenographic study of adult learning engagement in LEGO® Serious Play.* (Publication No.13808145) [Doctoral dissertation, Fielding Graduate University]. ProQuest Dissertations and Theses Publishing.

Cohen-Konrad, S. (2013). *Child and family practice: A relational perspective.* Oxford Publishing.

Dann, S. (2018). Facilitating co-creation experience in the classroom with LEGO® Serious Play. *Australasian Marketing Journal, 26,* 121–131.

Dykes, W. W. (2018). *Play well: Constructing creative confidence with LEGO® Serious Play* (Publication No. 10980351) [Doctoral dissertation, Fielding Graduate University]. ProQuest Dissertations and Theses Publishing.

Echterling, L. G., Presbury, J., & McKee, J. E. (2005). *Crisis intervention: Promoting resilience and resolution in troubled times.* Merrill/Prentice Hall.

Edmondson, A. C. (1999). Psychological safety and learning behavior in work teams. *Administrative Science Quarterly, 44*(2), 350–383.

Gauntlett, D. (2007). *Creative explorations: New approaches to identities and audiences.* Routledge.

Gauntlett, D. (2015). The LEGO® system as a tool for thinking, creativity, and changing the world. In D. Gauntlett: *Making media studies: The creativity turn in media and communications studies* (pp. 97–114). Peter Lang Publishing.

Grant, R. J., Stone, J., & Mellenthin, C. (Eds.) (2021). *Play therapy theories and perspectives: A collection of thoughts in the field* (pp. 198–206). Routledge.

Gray, P. (2009). Play as a foundation for hunter-gatherer social existence. *American Journal of Play*, 1, 476–522.

Harn, P. L. (2017). A preliminary study of the empowerment effects of strength-based LEGO® Serious Play on two Taiwanese adult survivors by earlier domestic violence. *Psychological Studies*, 62(2),142–151.

Harn, P. L. (2018). LEGO®-based clinical intervention with LEGO® Serious Play and Six Bricks for emotional regulation and cognitional reconstruction. *Examines Physical Medicine and Rehabilitation*, 1(3). EPMR.000515. 2018. doi:10.31031/EPMR.2018.01.000515.

Harn, P. L. & Hsiao, C. C. (2018). A preliminary study on LEGO®-based workplace stress reduction with Six Bricks and LEGO® Serious Play in Taiwan. *World Journal of Research and Review*, 6(1), 64–67.

Holliday, G., Statler, M., & Flanders, M. (2007). Developing practically wise leaders through serious play. *Consulting Psychology Journal*, 59, 126–134.

Huebner, A. J., Mancini, J. A., Wilcox, R. M., Grass, S. R., & Grass, G. A. (2007). Parental deployment and youth in military families: Exploring uncertainty and ambiguous loss. *Family Relations*, 56(2), 112–122.

James, A. (2015). *Innovative pedagogies series: Innovating in the creative arts with LEGO®*. Higher Education Academy.

Kees, M. & Rosenblum, K. (2015). Evaluation of a psychological health and resilience intervention for military spouses: A pilot study. *Psychological Services*, 12 (3), 222–230.

Kestly, T. A. (2014). *The interpersonal neurobiology of play*. W. W. Norton & Company.

Kristiansen, P. & Rasmussen, R. (2014). *Building a better business using the LEGO® Serious Play method*. Wiley.

LEGO® Foundation. (2018). *LEGO® play well report*. www.LEGO®foundation. com/media/1441/LEGO®-play-well-report-2018.pdf.

LEGO® Serious Play. (2010). Open source introduction to LEGO® Serious Play www.dropbox.com/s/8n2drwvqq5tzqdl/LSP_Open_Source.pdf?dl=0

Legoff, D. B., Gomez de la Cuesta, G., Kraus, G. W., & Baron-Cohen, S. (2014). *LEGO®-based therapy: How to build social competence through LEGO® based clubs for children with autism and related conditions*. Jessica Kingsley Publishers.

MacCormack, J. W. H., Hutchinson, L. A., & Matheson, N. L. (2015). An exploration of a LEGO® based social skills program for youth with autism spectrum disorder. *Exceptionality Education International*, 25, 13–32.

Mansfield, A. J., Kaufman, J. S., Marshall, S. W., Gaynes, B. N., Morrissey, J. P., & Engel, C. C. (2010). Deployment and the use of mental health service among U.S. Army wives. *The New England Journal of Medicine*, 362(2), 101–109.

McAuliffe, G. & Eriksen, K. (Eds.) (2011). *Handbook of counselor preparation: Constructivist, developmental and experiential approaches*. Sage.

McGuire, J. B., Paulus, C. J., & Quinn, L. (2015). *Mediated dialogue: Seeing your way through change*. Center for Creative Leadership.

Nerantzi, C. & James, A. (2019). *LEGO® for university learning: Inspiring academic practice in higher education*. 10.5281/zenodo.2813448. www.researchgate.net/publication/333844518_LEGO®R_for_university_learning_inspiring_academic_practice_in_higher_education.

Owens G., Granader, Y., Humphrey, A., & Baron-Cohen, S. (2008). LEGO® therapy and the social use of language programme: An evaluation of two social skills interventions for children with high functioning autism and Asperger Syndrome. *Journal of Autism Developmental Disorder*, 38(10),1944–1957.

Papert, S. (1999). *Papert on Piaget*. www.papert.org/articles/Papertonpiaget.html.

Papert, S. & Harel, I. (1991). Situating constructionism [Internet]. In Papert, S. & Harel, I. (Eds.), *Constructionism*. Ablex Publishing Corporation. www.papert.org/articles/SituatingConstructionism.html.

Peabody, M. A. (2015). Building with purpose: Using LEGO® Serious Play in play therapy supervision. *International Journal of Play Therapy*, 24(1), 30–40.

Peabody, M. A. & Noyes, S. (2017). Reflective boot camp: Adapting LEGO® Serious Play in higher education. *Reflective Practice: International and Multi-disciplinary Perspectives*, 18(2), 232–243.

Peabody, M. A. & Turesky, E. F. (2018). Shared leadership lessons: Adapting LEGO® Serious Play in higher education. *Journal of Management and Applied Research*, 5(4), 210–223.

Piaget, J. (1964). *The early growth of logic in the child*. Routledge.

Robertson, D. & Breen, B. (2013). *Brick by brick: How LEGO® rewrote the rules of innovation and conquered the global toy industry*. Crown Business: Random House.

Schaefer, C. E. (2003). *Play therapy with adults*. Wiley.

Schaefer, C. E. & Drewes, A. A. (Eds.) (2014). *The therapeutic powers of play: 20 core agents of change*, (2nd ed.), Wiley.

Statler, M., Heracleous, L., & Jacobs, C. D. (2011). Serious play as a practice of paradox. *Journal of Applied Behavioral Science*, 47(2), 236–256.

Sutton, J. (2012). When psychologists become builders. *The Psychologist*, 25(2). 600–603. https://thepsychologist.bps.org.uk/volume-25/edition-8/when-psychologists-become- builders.

Terr, L. (1999). *Beyond love and work: Why adults need to play*. Touchstone.

Thomsen, A. (2018). *Thera-Build*. Image.

Tulluck, D. (2020). *Brick-based counseling*. Youthlight, Inc.

Umhoefer, J. A., Peabody, M. A., & Stewart, A. L. (2015). Play therapy with military-connected children and families. In: D. A. Crenshaw & A. L. Stewart (Eds.), *Play therapy: A comprehensive guide to theory and practice* (pp. 385–399). Guilford.

Walsh A. (2019). Giving permission for adults to play. *The Journal of Play in Adulthood*. 1(1), 1–14.

Yalom, I. D. (1995). *The theory and practice of group psychotherapy* (4th ed.). Basic Books.

Yalom, I. D. & Leszcz, M. (2005). *The theory and practice of group psychotherapy* (5th ed.). Basic Books.

2 Humanistic Sandtray with Preadolescent Groups

Steven A. Armstrong, Ryan D. Foster, and Donna L. Hickman

Humanistic play therapists often provide interventions for children who are in the preoperational stage of cognitive development (ages 4–8). In child-centered play therapy (Landreth, 2012), therapists allow the child to lead and provide carefully selected, age-appropriate toys in a playroom designed to enhance fantasy and imaginative play. Child-centered play therapists "structure" the session by utilizing therapeutic toys carefully arranged and organized and by setting appropriate limits. The only direction that the therapist provides initially is to say, "You can play with any of the toys in this playroom in many of the ways you would like." This beginning statement places the responsibility on the child to decide and choose which toys to play with and how to use them. In child-centered *group* play therapy (Sweeney et al., 2014), two or three children enter the playroom together and play alongside or with the other children depending on their age and development.

By contrast, humanistic sandtray therapists deliver an intervention to children aged 10 and older as well as to adolescents and adults. The sandtray experience may be planned ahead or initiated by the therapist instead of leaving the decision to the child. Sandtray therapists provide sand trays, sand, and carefully selected miniatures so that clients can build or create worlds in the sand that represent *self*. According to Homeyer and Sweeney (2011), sandtray therapy is an "expressive and projective mode of psychotherapy involving the unfolding and processing of intra- and inter-personal issues through the use of specific sandtray materials as a nonverbal medium of communication" (p. 4). Like child-centered play therapy, sandtray therapists believe that this indirect and symbolic form of expression allows clients to experience and disclose underlying emotions and thoughts that might be too threatening to verbalize. When clients create scenes in the sand and tell therapists about their scenes, the miniatures they have chosen are metaphorical. In other words, the miniatures are *like* the clients, but they are *not* the clients, providing a safer psychological distance than talk therapy (Armstrong, 2008; Homeyer & Sweeney, 2017). In talk therapy, clients are expected to talk directly to the therapist about *self*. Many adolescent and adult clients struggle to feel and express emotions in talk therapy but are able to express the same emotions in the safety of sandtray therapy.

DOI: 10.4324/9781003094531-2

Humanistic sandtray therapists structure the sessions by using a prompt: "What I'd like you to do is create a scene of your life the way it is now. You may include people and experiences from the past and future but focus primarily on the present." Depending on the age of the client, this prompt may be more specific or modified to make it more concrete. For example, preadolescents may need a less global and more concrete prompt such as, "What I would like you to do is to make a scene or picture in the sand with these miniature figures that is about your family." Similar prompts also can be utilized when humanistic sandtray therapy is provided to a group of preadolescents. In individual and group therapy settings, therapists structure the initial phase of sandtray to help clients understand the scope and focus of the scene they will be creating.

Humanistic Sandtray Therapy

Humanistic sandtray therapy (HST; Armstrong, 2008) is a type of play therapy (Flahive & Ray, 2007; Homeyer & Sweeney, 2017) that "allows clients to express their inner worlds through symbol and metaphor" (Even & Armstrong, 2011, p. 395). Humanistic sandtray therapists facilitate a process of exploration grounded in and supported by a deep therapeutic relationship that focuses on here and now inner experiencing. For HST to be effective, it is essential for clients to experience themselves as being fully received by the therapist. According to Rogers (1961), this experience of being received means feeling fully understood and accepted.

HST is grounded in two schools of humanistic theory: person-centered and gestalt therapy. Both theories emphasize the importance of the therapeutic relationship, humanistic sandtray therapists believe that when they are able to establish a relationship that meets Rogers' (1957) six necessary and sufficient conditions, positive growth and change will result (see Table 2.1). Though it sounds straightforward enough, meeting Rogers' six conditions is difficult for therapists to achieve.

Therapists who want to develop the capacity to meet Rogers' six conditions must be engaged in a personal growth and awareness process in which they become increasingly more open to their own experiencing and develop the capacity to accept and allow all their own emotions into awareness (Rogers, 1961; Wilkins, 2010). Instead of a therapeutic role that is heavily focused on technique, diagnosis, or analysis, it is important for humanistic sandtray therapists to have the capacity to be fully present with clients in the moment. According to Bozarth (2001), therapists with unconditional positive self-regard (UPSR) are more able to be fully present because they have an increased capacity to allow all experiences (including negative and dysphoric ones) into awareness.

In addition to these demands on the person of the therapist, humanistic sandtray therapists facilitate a gestalt-oriented "phenomenological method of awareness in which perceiving, feeling, and acting are distinguished

Table 2.1 Carl Rogers' Six Conditions

Condition	Concept
Contact	Therapist makes initial, reciprocal psychological contact with the client
Client Incongruence	The client arrives to therapy in a vulnerable or anxious state
Congruence	Therapist remains authentic and genuine; "outward behavior is an accurate reflection of inner state" (Wilkins, 2010, p. 57)
Unconditional Positive Regard	Therapist's full acceptance of the client's person and experience
Empathy	Therapist's sensitive understanding of and communication about the client's internal experiencing and perception of the self, others, and their world
Client Receptivity to Facilitative Attitudes	The client must perceive and receive the therapist's psychological contact, congruence, unconditional positive regard, and empathy

Source: Adapted from The necessary and sufficient conditions of therapeutic personality change by C. R. Rogers, 1957, *Journal of Consulting Psychology, 21*(2), 95–103.

from interpreting and reshuffling pre-existing attitudes. Explanations and interpretations are considered less reliable than what is directly perceived and felt" (Yontef & Simkins, 1989, p. 323). Effective humanistic sandtray therapists focus on the inner experiencing of clients, place an emphasis on the here and now, and possess the ability to be fully present, accepting, and empathic. When therapists emphasize the inner experiencing of clients in the here and now, therapists must acquire the ability to gently guide clients into a descriptive process that avoids analysis and detailed story telling. Being fully present with clients in the here and now enhances the therapists' ability to connect to clients more deeply (Mearns & Cooper, 2005).

The Nature of Clients

Humanistic sandtray therapists believe that clients are born with the capacity to grow and develop into fully functioning beings if they receive consistent nurturing interaction from their caregivers (Greenspan & Shanker, 2004; Rogers, 1961; Wilkins, 2010). All clients are born with an actualizing tendency that propels them to growth and this process of becoming will proceed unless it is inhibited by a lack of support and affirmation. Clients also possess the capacity to be aware and choose. If they feel safe, valued, and accepted they will naturally experience and express a wide range of emotions and develop a sense of trust in their inner experiencing (Armstrong et al., 2016; Wilkins, 2010). HST allows clients to return to a long-forgotten sense of self with the capacity to complete their gestalts as moment-to-moment needs arise.

Maladjustment

Unfortunately, many children do not feel safe and accepted and thus may begin to doubt their own abilities and perceptions and become overly dependent on external validation. Wilkins (2010) noted that children are by nature vulnerable to criticism and negative appraisals of their worth. Wilkins stressed that children are so susceptible to invalidation diminishing their self-worth that one negative experience of criticism or negative appraisal can have a lasting effect. If children begin to doubt the accuracy of their perceptions and experience, they tend to begin to disregard and ignore their own experiencing and seek external validation and love. They begin to feel unbalanced in their perception of themselves and their environments.

Change

Regardless of theoretical orientation, the therapeutic relationship is the factor in psychotherapy that is most highly associated with positive client outcomes (Asay & Lambert, 2008; Frank & Frank, 1991; Hansen, 2005; Norcross & Wampold, 2011; Wampold & Bhati, 2004). In HST, the depth of the therapeutic relationship is regarded as the curative factor in therapy. The therapist does not try to change anything about the client. Change comes about when the therapist completely accepts the client, and the client enters into increased awareness and begins to accept themselves. Therefore, change in HST is paradoxical: clients change without *trying* to change themselves. As clients begin to change and move toward becoming more fully functioning people, they tend to become more open to increasing their awareness of how they respond to other people and their own emotions. This increased awareness allows clients to change self-defeating habits that have hindered the quality of their lives.

Phases of a Sandtray Session

Phase One: Preparation and Setup

It takes considerable preparation to conduct sandtray therapy and this begins with the acquisition of materials: sand, a sand tray, and miniatures. Aspiring sandtray therapists can acquire these online but there are advantages to shopping for miniatures in person. We have found used miniatures in toy stores that are far less expensive than shopping for fancy figures at

specialty stores. Homeyer and Sweeney (2017) recommended that therapists have a minimum of 300 miniature figures, but they noted that 500 or
1000 will provide clients a more facilitative number of miniatures; readers
are directed to their book for explicit suggestions on categories of miniatures, type of sand, and size of sand trays.

Phase Two: Introduction and Scene Creation

If clients have not had the opportunity to become familiar with the miniatures, the sand, and the tray, it is helpful for them to spend time surveying
and touching these media. Preadolescents may need only 5–10 minutes to feel
comfortable with the materials, but adults may require more time. Adults
take much more time looking at and touching the miniatures so that they
may find a figure that captures exactly what they want to represent.

As mentioned earlier, with adolescents and adults, a prompt is typically
provided before clients create their scenes: "What I'd like you to do is
create a scene of your life the way it is now. You may include people and
experiences from the past and future but focus primarily on the present."
When clients are choosing miniatures and beginning to build their scenes,
the HST therapist usually does not talk or intrude in the process but the
therapist is attentive (in a subtle way) and available if the client verbalizes
something during the scene creation phase of the session.

Phase Three: Processing

Once clients have finished creating their scenes in the sand, the processing
phase of sandtray therapy begins. In HST, many adolescent and adult clients
are willing to explore metaphors and related issues openly in their sandtray
scenes, which can elicit underlying emotions. If clients do not trust the
therapist to a significant degree, they are not ready for this kind of experience
but if the quality and depth of the therapeutic relationship has provided a
secure enough base for clients to engage in an honest process of self-
exploration of the metaphors in their trays, many clients are willing to allow
underlying emotions and issues to come to the surface. We believe that clients
are experiencing beings by nature who have been encouraged to lean on
external sources of validation (Wilkins, 2010). However, if clients are willing
to reconnect to themselves on a deeper level, they can continue the process of
becoming a fully functioning person that they were meant to experience. The
symbolic nature of sandtray therapy combined with the safety, understanding, and acceptance of the therapist can give clients courage to experience and accept their emotions on a deeper level.

Homeyer and Sweeney (2017) described the processing phase as one in
which clients guide the therapist into the clients' worlds. However, humanistic sandtray therapists emphasize the here and now inner experiencing
of clients more than other approaches (Hanson, 2005). Clients assume a

major role in the processing of the tray, but the therapist structures this part of the session. For example, as clients create their scenes in the tray, many of them begin to experience emotions and frequently exhibit non-verbal expressions of emotion *prior to* the beginning of the processing phase of sandtray. When the client sits down next to the therapist to begin the processing phase of the session, the therapist will typically focus on the client's inner experiencing. The therapist might say, "It looks like creating the scene has brought some sadness to the surface for you."

Humanistic sandtray therapists strive to find the optimal balance between focusing on the sandtray scene and the inner experiencing of the client. When clients indicate nonverbally that they are experiencing an emotion in the moment, the therapist may explore their emotions for several minutes before returning to the scene in the tray. When clients are explaining the meaning and significance of their scenes to the therapist, the therapist communicates empathy and support nonverbally and may choose not to respond verbally to the client. This oscillation is typical of the processing phase in HST.

When clients are experiencing emotional pain in the middle of a sand-tray session – which is quite common – the therapist may process this experience for 10–15 minutes without focusing on other parts of the sandtray scene. In other words, humanistic sandtray therapists believe that an in-depth process of exploration, expression, and experiencing of the client's emotions in the session facilitates growth and awareness in a pow-erful and possibly transformative way. Humanistic sandtray therapists need to be highly skilled in noticing, sensing, and responding to nonverbal expressions of emotion in the session because most clients do not verbally express emotion in the moment. When clients are experiencing emotion in the here and now, instead of telling the therapist that they are feeling sad, angry, or afraid, they show it nonverbally in their facial expressions, tone of voice, and bodily movements. Most adolescent and adult clients enga-ging in sandtray therapy stop and control expressions of emotion while they are experiencing it. They are afraid of experiencing emotion fully and restrict it to some degree by increasing tension in their bodies.

Phase Four: Clean-up and Documentation

After processing the tray, the session is completed, and the client exits the room. The dismantling of the scene should be done after the client leaves the room. This delay allows the client to retain the image of the scene in his or her mind (Homeyer & Sweeney, 2017). It is common for therapists to take a picture of clients' sandtrays for documentation.

Group Work and Sandtray

HST can be used with groups in a variety of ways with a wide range of ages and issues. It can be used occasionally as an activity in a therapy or process group, frequently or exclusively in a preadolescent or adolescent therapy group (Flahive & Ray, 2007; Shen & Armstrong, 2008), or regularly in a counselor training or supervision group (Armstrong, 2008). HST procedures can be adapted for groups of preadolescents, adolescents, and adults. For the purposes of this chapter, we will focus on HST with preadolescents. In addition to a description of a rationale and procedures for providing HST to preadolescents in groups, we will provide a case example of HST with a group of sixth grade boys.

Preadolescent Groups

In HST with groups of preadolescents, group therapists are aware that members may not be able to process their sandtray scenes like older adolescents and adults. Humanistic therapists believe that preadolescents are born with an actualizing tendency that makes them capable of self-direction in a climate of freedom, acceptance, and emotional support. Draper, Ritter, and Willingham (2003) described the use of sandtray therapy in a group with preadolescents as an intervention in which "group members build small worlds with miniature figures in individual trays of sand and share about their worlds as they are willing" (p. 244). Bratton and Ferebee (1999) stated that using sandtray in a group gives preadolescents "opportunities to change perceptions about self, others and the world" (p. 193). Because preadolescents are transitioning from concrete to abstract thinking and may still have difficulty verbalizing their thoughts and feelings, using sandtray in groups can allow them to use a more concrete and safe mode of expression (Flahive & Ray, 2007). Draper et al. (2003) added that children in this age group can benefit from a "modality that is not completely dependent on verbalization" (p. 245).

Flahive and Ray (2007) developed procedures for the delivery of group sandtray therapy with preadolescents. They recommended limiting the size of preadolescent sandtray therapy groups to four group members and meeting for one hour. The small size of the group allows each group member to have enough time to share their scenes with the whole group. They also recommended detailed procedures for setting up the sandtray room including trays and miniatures and providing detailed instructions to the group members. Flahive and Ray suggested that the sandtray room be set up with four 20-inch plastic trays and shelves or tables to display miniatures. As Homeyer and Sweeney (2011) recommended, if possible, the miniatures should include people, animals, buildings, vehicles, fences, natural items, and fantasy and spiritual-mystical figures and objects. Flahive and Ray (2007) recommended that participants be told to look at the miniatures on the shelves or tables. In addition, they provided the following instructions:

> I would like you to build a scene of _____ (the selected topic as described earlier) in your own sandtray by using the sand and the miniatures

there. You may build your sandtray scene in any way you like and use as many miniatures as you would like. When you are working on building your scene, I will sit here quietly. Let me know when you are finished.

Shen and Armstrong (2008) recommended using specific topics for each preadolescent group session. For example, working with groups of pre-adolescent girls that were heterogeneous by race, the authors suggested in one group session that the girls build a scene of themselves and their friends. In another session, because the purpose of the sandtray therapy group was to help seventh grade girls improve self-esteem, the group leader instructed the group members to create a scene about how they felt about their physical appearance.

After group members create their scenes, the group leader invites the group members to share their sandtray scenes. The group leader might say, "What would you like to share about your sandtray scene with us? There may be something there that you do not want to share, and that is fine. You may share it in any way you like." (Shen & Armstrong, 2008, p. 127). When group members share their scenes, the leader might reflect feelings, ask if the preadolescent can tell more about their scene or ask about certain miniatures that seem to have significance. In addition, the group leader typically uses group skills such as linking to normalize responses and feelings to promote universality and cohesiveness.

Group Phases

HST can be used across group phases typically known as forming, storming, norming, performing (Tuckman, 1965), and adjourning (Tuckman & Jensen, 1977). During the forming stage, HST can act as an exercise to introduce members to each other and begin to form individual and group objectives. A useful prompt during this phase in a preadolescent group might be, "Create a world that helps others know who you are. You could include likes, dislikes, wishes, hopes, and challenges."

During the storming stage, HST can be used to assist members to communicate intragroup conflicts and head toward resolution. One prompt might be, "Build a scene in the sand that shows how you see you and your group members." Using a prompt like this can be an effective way to bring group conflicts into the open view of the leader and the members in order to work toward a more honest group dynamic. HST during this stage can also act to propel group members toward increased group cohesion.

HST takes on a slightly different role in the norming stage. Group members here know each other quite well, have worked through major member to member or member to leader conflicts successfully, and have found trust in the group process. They feel an established set of group rules and roles and relate more readily and openly. HST during this stage acts as a partner to these group processes. One prompt that can be responsive to the dynamics during the norming stage is, "Using any of the miniatures you'd like, make a scene that depicts your favorite problem-solving tools."

The performing stage is where the outcome-oriented work takes place. In this way, HST can be used as an intervention itself to help members work out intragroup conflict or even to engage members in peer support. For example, group members could be prompted to create a scene in the sandtray about how they see each other's worlds. This prompt can act as a way to continue to solidify group cohesion and relationship between group members, as well as allowing group members to demonstrate the growth that they have seen in each other.

Finally, in the adjourning stage, HST can be a powerful mechanism to assist in the termination process as a way to reflect on members' group experiences or to demonstrate optimism, hope, and growth in the future. A prompt such as, "Make a scene in the sandtray that shows how you have seen yourself change" can be one way of adjuncting termination. Another prompt might be, "Make a scene that shows others how you feel about ending the group." There are a number of meaningful ways to integrate HST into the termination phase of group counseling.

Research on Humanistic Sandtray Therapy

There is a scant amount of research on sandtray and its sibling, sandplay therapy. Most research has been based in case study research, particularly with sandplay therapy (Foo et al., 2020; Mitchell & Friedman, 1994), although a small number of studies have used quantitative designs. Because HST is a relatively newer model of sandtray therapy, we will discuss what we know based on emerging research.

Lyles and Homeyer (2015) noted in their case studies of using HST with adoptive families that HST appeared to be an effective approach to helping their clients attune empathically with each other and provide a healing space for attachment. Eberts and Homeyer (2015) processed sandtrays with each other, one from an Adlerian approach and the other a gestalt approach. They reported their experiences as the facilitator and in the client role and reflected that each approach to sandtray seemed to bring about change in themselves. Armstrong et al., (2015) described two case studies of a school counselor using HST and reported that it resulted in students' increased abilities to express emotion more openly. Teachers reporting a few months later supported these notable changes in behavior in their classrooms, as well.

There are three quantitative studies to date exploring the use of HST in groups. Earlier, we described Flahive and Ray's (2007) approach. They used an experimental design with 56 preadolescents – 28 in the experimental and

28 in the control group – to investigate the impact of HST on disruptive classroom behaviors. Using the BASC-TRS, they found statistically significant differences with medium effect sizes in three areas: the Behavior Symptom Index, the Behavior Problem Scale, and the Externalizing Behavior Problem Scale. They concluded that their results suggested that HST had a "positive therapeutic impact on preadolescents with behavioral difficulties" (p. 379).

Shen and Armstrong (2008), whose approach we also described previously, carried out a quasi-experimental study in which they used a treatment and control group but did not use random assignment. Using the Self-Perception Profile for Children (SPPC) to measure self-esteem with groups of young adolescent females, they found statistically significant interactions with medium to large effect sizes on five of the six subscales. They concluded that HST appeared to improve self-esteem with groups of young adolescent girls. More information about the SPPC can be found online.

Swank and Lenes (2013) used an approach similar to Flahive and Ray (2007) and Shen and Armstrong (2008), but notably used HST with groups of adolescent females in an alternative school. In this phenomenological qualitative study, Swank and Lenes (2013) provided weekly group sandtray therapy to 21 participants over five weeks. After conclusion of the five-week group counseling program, members participated in semi-structured interviews as well as focus groups. Themes that emerged included self-expression, development of insight, growth opportunities, hope, and group dynamics. Self-expression captured participants finding that sandtray helped them to depict thoughts, feelings, and experiences that were difficult to put into words. Development of insight indicated participants' increasing understanding about self, others, and their contexts. Growth opportunities revealed that participants were able to put expression and insight into behavioral change. Hope captured participants' increased senses of internal loci of control and self-esteem. Finally, group dynamics was reflective of participants finding peer support and opportunities to listen and feel heard within the group dynamics by sharing and seeing other group members' sandtrays.

In summary, HST has supportive research that highlights its utility in group counseling environments, particularly with children and adolescents. However, a call for more quantitative and qualitative research into the structure, function, and processes that are practiced by humanistic sandtray therapists is imperative. Following is a case example that underscores the power of HST.

Preadolescent Case Example

Lucas was a 12-year-old, sixth grade boy who was referred by his teacher to the first author (S.A.) for group counseling in his school. His teacher was concerned about Lucas fitting in better because he had moved to the school at the beginning of sixth grade and had not been able to develop any real friendships with other students. In addition, he frequently misbehaved in class to get attention. His group consisted of six boys who met once a week during school hours. The group was semi-structured and included activities and topics for each meeting. Sandtray was one of the interventions introduced to the group after the boys had met for six sessions.

In the sandtray group session, the boys were asked to make a scene in their tray about their families. The boys were encouraged to be honest about things they liked and disliked at home. Lucas was an only child, and he created a scene that had a few objects including three people, a dog, a house, and some greenery. Most of the boys shared about their sandtray scene but none of them were required to talk about anything they did not want to share.

When it was Lucas' turn to talk about his scene, he began to talk seriously about some of the problems he was having with his mother and stepfather. Until now, Lucas had participated appropriately in the group, but he had never experienced any emotion when he shared. As he talked about how his stepfather treated him, Lucas focused on the figure he had chosen for himself and told the boys that when his stepfather was really mad, he would lock Lucas out of the house and make him spend the night outside. Lucas' mother objected to this type of punishment but was afraid to intervene.

As Lucas shared about spending the night outside, he began to cry. He told the other boys that he had been cold and afraid. As the leader, I empathized and reflected how scary it must be for Lucas to spend the night outside alone. After a few minutes, Lucas stopped crying. Initially, the other boys were quiet due to the seriousness of Lucas' situation and the sadness he expressed. Once Lucas stopped crying and began to feel a little better, several of the boys were very supportive and said that the stepfather should never have done that. As the boys left the group that day, it appeared that something in the group had shifted. The boys walked out with Lucas and continued to talk to him as they walked down the hall. In the weeks after this session, I noticed that outside of the group, Lucas was hanging out with three of the boys and seemed to be a part of their group. When I talked to Lucas' teacher, she reported that Lucas seemed happier and now had some friends in the class.

*Due to various circumstances that cannot be covered in this chapter, a child protection report was not made in this situation.

Conclusion

To summarize, HST is a creative and effective therapeutic approach to use with groups of preadolescents. Emerging research, as well as our clinical experiences, demonstrate that HST can be used with groups of pre-adolescents who are struggling with a variety of issues and can allow clients freedom to increase self and other awareness, gain understanding, and engage in paradoxical change. As an integrative approach built upon person-centered and gestalt frameworks, HST provides an empathic, compassionate, connecting, and freeing space as either an adjunct for group work or as a standalone group modality.

References

Armstrong, S. A. (2008). *Sandtray therapy: A humanistic approach*. Ludic Press.

Armstrong, S. A., Brown, T., & Foster, R. D. (2015). Humanistic sandtray therapy with preadolescents. *Journal of Child and Adolescent Counseling*, 1(1), 17–26. doi:10.1080/23727810.2015.1023167.

Armstrong, S. A., Foster, R. D., Brown, T., & Davis, J. (2016). Humanistic sandtray therapy with children and adults. In E. Leggett & J. Boswell (Eds.), *Directive play therapy: Theories and techniques* (pp. 217–254). Springer.

Asay, T. P. & Lambert, M. J. (2008). The empirical case for the common factors in therapy: Quantitative findings. In M. A. Hubble, B. L. Duncan, & S. D. Miller (Eds.), *The heart and soul of change: What works in therapy* (pp. 23–55). American Psychological Association.

Bozarth, J. D. (2001). Congruence: A special way of being. In G. Wyatt (Ed.), *Congruence. Rogers' therapeutic conditions: Evolution, theory and practice* (pp. 184–199). PCCS Books.

Bratton, S. C. & Ferebee, K. W. (1999). The use of structured expressive art activities in group activity therapy with preadolescents. In D. S. Sweeney & L. E. Homeyer (Eds.), *The handbook of group play therapy* (pp. 192–214). Jossey-Bass.

Draper, K., Ritter, K. B., & Willingham, E. U. (2003). Sand tray group counseling with adolescents. *Journal for Specialists in Group Work*, 28(3), 244–260. doi:10.1177/0193392203252030.

Eberts, S. & Homeyer, L. (2015). Processing sand trays from two theoretical perspectives: Gestalt and Adlerian. *International Journal of Play Therapy*, 24(3), 134–150. doi:10.1037/a0039392.

Even, T. A. & Armstrong, S. A. (2011). Sandtray for early recollections with children (SERCh) in Adlerian play therapy. *Journal of Individual Psychology*, 67, 391–407.

Flahive, M. & Ray, D. (2007). Effect of group sandtray therapy with preadolescents in a school setting. *Journal for Specialists in Group Work*, 32, 362–382. doi:10.1080/01933920701476706.

Foo, M., Freedle, L.R., Sani, R., & Fonda, G. (2020). The effect of sandplay therapy on the thalamus in the treatment of generalized anxiety disorder: A case report. *International Journal of Play Therapy*, 29(4), 191–200. doi:10.1037/pla0000137.

Frank, J. D. & Frank, J. B. (1991). *Persuasion and healing* (3rd ed.). Johns Hopkins University Press.

Greenspan, S. I. & Shanker, S. G. (2004). *The first idea: How symbols, language, and intelligence evolved from our primate ancestors to modern humans*. Da Capo Press.

Hansen, J. T. (2005). The devaluation of inner subjective experiences by the counseling profession: A plea to reclaim the essence of the profession. *Journal of Counseling & Development*, 83, 406–415. https://doi.org/10.1002/j.1556-6678. 2005.tb00362.x.

Homeyer, L. & Sweeney, D. (2011). *Sandtray therapy: A practical manual* (2nd ed.). Routledge.

Homeyer, L. & Sweeney, D. (2017). *Sandtray therapy: A practical manual* (3rd ed.). Routledge.

Landreth, G. (2012). *Play therapy: The art of the relationship* (3rd ed.). Routledge.

Lyles, M. & Homeyer, L. (2015). The use of sandtray therapy with adoptive families. *Adoption Quarterly*, 18(1), 67–80. https://doi.org/10.1080/10926755. 2014.945704.

Mearns, D. & Cooper, M. (2005). *Working at relational depth in counselling and psychotherapy*. Sage.

Mitchell, R. R. & Friedman, H. S. (1994). *Sandplay: Past, present and future*. Taylor & Francis/Routledge.

Norcross, J. C. & Wampold, B. E. (2011). Evidence-based therapy relationships: Research conclusions and clinical practices. *Psychotherapy*, 48, 98–102. doi:10.1037/a0022161.

Rogers, C. R. (1957). The necessary and sufficient conditions of therapeutic personality change. *Journal of Consulting Psychology*, 21(2), 95–103. doi:10.1037/h0045357.

Rogers, C. R. (1961). *On becoming a person*. Houghton Mifflin.

Shen, Y. & Armstrong, S. A. (2008). Impact of group sandtray therapy on the self-esteem of young adolescent girls. *Journal for Specialists in Group Work*, 33, 118–137. doi:10.1080/01933920801977397.

Swank, J. M. & Lenes, E. A. (2013). An exploratory inquiry of sandtray group experiences with adolescent females in an alternative school. *Journal for Specialists in Group Work*, 38(4), 330–348. doi:10.1080/01933922.2013.835013.

Sweeney, D. S., Baggerly, J. N., & Ray, D. (2014). *Group play therapy: A dynamic approach*. Routledge.

Tuckman, B. (1965). Developmental sequence in small groups. *Psychological Bulletin*, 63(6), 384–399. doi:10.1037/h0022100.

Tuckman, B. W. & Jensen, M. A. C. (1977). Stages of small-group development revisited. *Group & Organization Management*, 2(4), 419–427. doi:10.1177%2F105960117700200404.

Wampold, B. E. & Bhati, K. S. (2004). Attending to the omissions: A historical examination of evidence-based practice movements. *Professional Psychology: Research and Practice*, 35, 563–570. doi:10.1037/0735-7028.35.6.563.

Wilkins, P. (2010). *Person-centred therapy: 100 key points*. Routledge.

Yontef, G. M. & Simkin, J. S. (1989). Gestalt therapy. In R. J. Corsini & D. Wedding (Eds.), *Current psychotherapies* (4th ed.) (pp. 323–361). F. E. Peacock.

3 The *Caped Crusaders*

Using Superheroes in a Play Therapy Group for Adolescents

Sophia Ansari

"A long time ago in a galaxy far, far away...." are words that instantly transport us into a world where cultural icons represent the fear, grief, and courage within us. Storytelling has always been an integral part of human culture and learning. Legends, stories, and parables have been passed down from generation to generation as a means of teaching important life lessons and values. Perhaps one of the most magical aspects of *Harry Potter* is that research has shown that reading *Harry Potter* may increase tolerance and empathy in its readers (Hsu et al., 2014; Vezzali et al., 2014). Superhero and fantasy stories offer us a realm of experience in which we can share the emotions of our favorite fictional characters while also replenishing crucial psychological energy that we use trying to cope with real life. Through the blending of narrative therapy, expressive arts, and play therapy, individuals can better understand themselves and how to navigate the world around them. Although younger children might be unable to verbalize their thoughts and feelings, they often gain insight as they identify with their favorite superheroes. It is through this filter of fiction that we can inspire, support, and instill the spirit of growth and resilience and this can be especially true in group work.

Overview

The *Caped Crusaders* is a group created by this author for adolescents to enhance positive change after adversity. It was established to meet the needs of children diagnosed with Post-Traumatic Stress Disorder (PTSD) who have experienced community violence such as bullying, gun violence, and gang violence. The *Caped Crusaders* provides a safe superhero lair; a space to deepen connection between group members and celebrate their strengths (superpowers). The focus of the group is to work to facilitate post-traumatic growth and resilience using the theoretical frameworks of Positive Psychology and Acceptance and Commitment Therapy. Both emphasize the importance of utilizing strengths to accomplish goals and exploring values to move toward finding meaning and purpose (Ciarrochi et al., 2013).

DOI: 10.4324/9781003094531-3

A typical group is closed, runs for 8 weeks, and can be modified to serve young children as well as adults. Members of the group also participate in weekly individual therapy to expand on individual and group treatment goals. Geek artifacts such as comic books, movies, and video games are utilized to help group members identify their personal strengths (super-powers), positive relationships with others (sidekicks), engage in mindfulness practices (elixir against the rumination monsters), and compassion for self and others (Kryptonite against self-criticism and self-isolation).

Superheroes are an essential component in *Caped Crusaders* groups. Superhero stories provide models of coping with trauma and adversity. Superheroes inspire us to find meaning in loss. Through identifying which superhero narratives motivate our clients and which themes are present in their play, we can better understand their relationships, battles (both internal and external), and how they overcome challenges. In addition to utilizing superhero stories, other mediums are also implemented in the groups such as cooperative video game play and tabletop games to increase social skills and enhance positive relationships. This concept was largely inspired by the Geek Therapy model, founded by Josué Cardona. Geek Therapy integrates evidence-based practices with geek culture and asserts that "the best way to understand each other, and ourselves, is through the media we care about" (Cardona, 2020, p. 15). Clinicians and educators use the child's interests to deepen connection and rapport while also utilizing the therapeutic power of storytelling. Cardona emphasizes that if it matters to our clients, it should matter to us (Cardona, 2020).

Research and Theory

Trauma is part of many superhero origin stories. These events fundamentally set them on a new path – to right the wrongs and protect others from experiencing the same pain and loss they suffered. This resolve to rely on inner strengths and find meaning and purpose is related to the concept of post-traumatic growth (PTG). Post-traumatic growth and resilience are often used interchangeably but they are two different concepts. Resilience is one's ability to adapt or "bounce back" from stress and trauma (Southwick et al., 2014). A resilient individual possesses a higher level of coping but may still experience challenges. Some individuals have a difficult time recovering from the traumatic event. This can trigger depression, anxiety, maladaptive coping skills, and can challenge their core beliefs. Post-traumatic growth involves finding meaning and purpose after trauma, where making sense of one's circumstances may lead to growth and positive change. Individuals work to reconstruct core beliefs about themselves and their worldview (Tedeschi et al., 2018). This positive mental shift can be a challenging journey because these thought patterns and behaviors were not present prior to the traumatic event. A number of factors can pave a path to the development of PTG: positive relationships with others, focusing on strengths, finding meaning in painful experiences, cognitive restructuring of one's worldview, and self-compassion and mindfulness practices (Germer & Barnhofer, 2017; Tedeschi et al., 2018).

Individuals often need assistance from other people, and superheroes are no different. Superheroes like Captain Marvel, Wonder Woman, and Thor are certainly formidable and mighty, but still count on their trusty teams (sidekicks and allies) to help them on difficult quests. Social support is an important predictor of mental health outcomes in children and adolescents. Research has suggested that social support fosters positive change in the aftermath of trauma and adversity by helping to facilitate cognitive processing, promote healthy coping strategies, and adaptation which can lead to PTG (Prati & Pietrantoni, 2009). It is within these safe spaces that individuals with shared experiences can form bonds of trust and healing while imparting wisdom gained from their own origin stories.

Often when individuals hear the word "superpower", they think of Superman, who can fly faster than the speed of light and absorb the power of the sun. While adolescents might be lacking in abilities such as superhuman strength, invulnerability, and X-ray vision, they do possess their own unique "superpowers" that are core to who they are. Like Superman, individuals can possess the superpowers of humility, honesty, perseverance, and bravery. These superpowers exist within all people in the form of character strengths which can be thought of as the best qualities in human beings (Niemiec, 2017).

Character strengths research was championed by Peterson and Seligman (2004) who outlined their groundbreaking study in the book titled, *Character Strengths and Virtues: A Handbook and Classification.* The researchers identified 24-character strengths. These strengths exist in all people in varying degrees. Individuals (ages 10 and up) can take the free VIA Survey at www.viacharacter.org to identify their unique character strengths profile. The top five strengths of the profile represent an individual's signature strengths. These strengths are essential to who the person is as they are expressed more effortlessly and naturally than the other strengths (Niemiec, 2017). Research has shown that identifying and applying signature strengths enhances well-being, engagement, and greater life satisfaction (Gander et al., 2012; MacConville, 2012).

For people who have experienced trauma and adversity, focusing on strengths can be exceedingly difficult. Individuals tend to see themselves as weak or broken. By utilizing a strengths-based perspective, survivors can see themselves as the heroes of their stories and move towards healing and recovery. Ansari and Scott (2019) discussed how to incorporate superheroes with strengths-based play therapy. By identifying strengths in oneself and others (favorite superheroes and heroes in everyday life), adolescents can tap into their inner powers to overcome adversity and flourish into beings far more epic than Superman.

The prevailing theme in Star Wars, it turns out, is self-compassion and mindfulness. The philosophies of the Jedi are centered on striving to be in the present moment, to care for oneself, and cultivate the Force which binds Jedi together. Self-compassion and mindfulness practices help build resilience by allowing us to check in with ourselves and then answer with a nurtured response. In the film *Star Wars: Episode I – The Phantom Menace* Qui-Gon Jinn directs Obi-Wan, "Don't center on your anxieties, Obi-Wan. Keep your concentration here and now, where it belongs" (Lucas, 1999, 0:03:15). This gem of wisdom signifies that using the Force requires living in the now. Mindfulness asks the question, *"What am I experiencing?"* (Germer & Barnhofer, 2017). It requires paying attention in a particular way; on purpose, in the present moment and non-judgmentally (Kabat-Zinn, 2009).

Research has shown engaging in mindfulness and self-compassion practices offers a range of social, cognitive, physical, and emotional benefits for adolescents (Bluth & Eisenlohr-Moul, 2017). Mindfulness can help individuals break free from the loops of negative thinking (rumination). Essentially, it means we can call upon our "Spidey" senses to pay attention to what we are doing and gives us room to respond to our feelings or respond to what is happening rather than just to react to them. Being rooted in the present moment allows one to escape the traps of experiential avoidance. Experiential avoidance is an attempt to suppress unwanted thoughts, feelings, memories, and bodily sensations (Hayes et al., 1999). This can be illustrated by our favorite supervillains (i.e., Darth Vader) who use this negative coping mechanism as a shield from experiencing pain, fear, and sadness (Ansari & Scott, 2019).

If mindfulness asks, *"What am I experiencing?"* then self-compassion asks, *"What do I need?"* (Germer & Barnhofer, 2017). Compassion is defined as the concern for the alleviation of suffering for self and others (Neff, 2011). Compassion can help us notice positive moments in life and can ease our internal threat system (Germer & Neff, 2015). Neff (2011) identified that self-compassion has three components: self-kindness, common humanity, and mindfulness.

- Self-kindness involves being kind to yourself instead of judgmental or critical. It is about speaking to yourself the way you would speak to a loved one. It is the healing potion to self-criticism.
- Recognition of a common humanity focuses on the interconnectedness between us all and the shared human experience rather than looking at our experiences as one of a kind. It is the healing potion to self-isolation.
- Mindfulness involves recognizing our suffering. By being mindful of our own pain we are giving ourselves space to respond to that pain rather than react to it. Mindfulness is the healing potion to combat self-absorption.

The three components of self-compassion are evident in the world of superheroes. Superheroes must take care of themselves first before they can help others (self-kindness). They must work with humans and other superheroes to bring about justice (common humanity). And they must learn to be present in the now rather than be consumed by their traumatic origins and experiences (mindfulness).

Several programs have been built to teach self-compassion to adolescents in recent years. The *Caped Crusaders* group curriculum implements the principles and practices of the empirically supported program titled, *Making Friends with Yourself* (MFY). This program was created by Karen Bluth and Lorraine Hobbs who adapted MFY from the Mindful Self-Compassion program for adults (Bluth, 2017). An adolescent typically possesses enough of a developed self-concept to be able to achieve the self-reflection needed for self-compassion. It is during these formative years that self-concept becomes much more differentiated and adolescents start to compare their real selves to their ideal selves which can lead to depression and anxiety. Teaching adolescents the power of self-compassion buffers this process. While they may still feel insecure and experience the typical emotional ups and downs, they can learn to be a good friend to themselves in the midst of difficult feelings. Studies have shown that self-compassion practices in adolescents reduces depression, anxiety, eating disorders, suicidal ideation, and increases academic motivation, resilience, and well-being (Bluth & Eisenlohr-Moul, 2017; Bluth et al., 2015; Neff & McGehee, 2010). Self-compassion practices assist individuals in supporting their imperfections as opposed to valuing "perfection". Therefore, self-compassion is a much more stable resource for adolescents than self-esteem work. When someone is a friend to themselves, everywhere they go, they have a supportive inner voice there to support and encourage them. Self-compassion is the ultimate superpower!

Group Example and Interventions

The following are some interventions and practices utilized in the *Caped Crusaders* curriculum that focus on elements key to facilitating PTG such as: enhancing positive relationships, identifying and applying strengths, and practicing self-compassion. Table 3.1 provides a brief overview of the group curriculum.

Superhero Team: A Forcefield of Character Strengths

The purpose of this activity is to highlight each group members' unique abilities, strengths (superpowers), and illustrate a visual of the support system (sidekicks and allies) the group provides. The activity begins with identifying superhero teams. Many adolescents will often list X-Men, Justice League, Fantastic Four, Teen Titans, The Avengers, Teenage Mutant Ninja Turtles, The Defenders, and Guardians of the Galaxy as dynamic superhero teams. The following question may then be presented to the

Table 3.1 The *Caped Crusaders* Group Curriculum

Purpose: To enhance positive change and well-being after trauma and adversity. Group members will cultivate healthy, positive, and genuine relationships with themselves and others.
Group Length: 90 minutes
Group Size: 4–6 members
Number of group facilitators: 2 (recommended)

Week	Goal	Materials Needed
1	Discuss group norms, identify strengths to foster a sense of common humanity that will help group members feel validated, understood, and part of a larger community.	• VIA Character Strengths profile for each group member • sand tray, superhero miniatures • media such as film, comic books, etc. to utilize in strengths spotting exercise • large sheet of paper for superhero shield, markers/pens • Sorting Hat*
2	Integrate interpersonal mindfulness and self-compassion with open sharing and processing of experiences to guide group members on their journey to well-being.	• paper and pen for self-compassion letter • comic books/media to demonstrate self-compassion and mindfulness themes (examples: *Star Wars, Doctor Who, Spider-Man, Ms. Marvel, Iron Fist, Steven Universe*) • self-compassion/mindfulness scripts and audio • Sorting Hat*
3	Identify strengths and feelings about self to increase positive feelings about self. Provide a visual metaphor to illustrate mindfulness.	• self-compassion potion: salt, colored chalk, paper plates, funnels, plastic potion bottles (notecard to write which color represents each signature strength) • mindful jar: mason jar/plastic water bottle, glitter glue, water, food coloring. Mindful script from: https://www.mindful.org/how-to-create-a-glitter-jar-for-kids/ • mindfulness and self-compassion examples from *Star Wars* and other media • Sorting Hat*
4	Introduction to ACT core principles. Learn psychological skills to change relationship with thoughts and feelings and set goals to move toward values.	• finger traps and film clip of the Devil's Snare from *Harry Potter and the Philosopher's Stone* (to demonstrate metaphor for experiential avoidance) • media to demonstrate ACT core principles (for example: *My Hero Academia, The Hunger Games, Lord of the Rings, Inside Out*) • "Face your monsters" activity: shrinky dinks paper, sharpies, markers, oven (used by clinician in between sessions) • Sorting Hat*

Purpose: To enhance positive change and well-being after trauma and adversity. Group members will cultivate healthy, positive, and genuine relationships with themselves and others.
Group Length: 90 minutes
Group Size: 4–6 members
Number of group facilitators: 2 (recommended)

Week	Goal	Materials Needed
5	Introduction to ACT core principles. Learn psychological skills to change relationship with thoughts and feelings and set goals to move toward values.	• completed shrinky dinks monsters/villains • clay or play-doh for superhero gadgets • media to demonstrate ACT core principles (for example: *My Hero Academia, The Hunger Games, Lord of the Rings, Inside Out*) • Sorting Hat*
6	Introduction to ACT core principles. Learn psychological skills to change relationship with thoughts and feelings and set goals to move toward values.	• sand tray and miniatures for group tray • ACT values worksheet • media to demonstrate ACT core principles (for example: *My Hero Academia, The Hunger Games, Lord of the Rings, Inside Out*) • Sorting Hat*
7	Cooperative video game play to provide an opportunity to build social skills, build a community together, explore together, engage in strengths spotting, and overcome obstacles together.	• building prompts given by group facilitator/s • video game of group facilitator's choice (example: Minecraft™) • Sorting Hat*
8	Create a visual representation of growth, the acceptance of change, and the power of resilience.	• broken pottery or blank puzzle pieces, broken toys, or LEGO® bricks, markers/sharpies, glue, gold leaf, or gold glitter glue

Note: *At the conclusion of each group session, members are to draw a strength from the *Harry Potter* Sorting Hat. Group members are instructed to use this strength in a new way, each day for a week and process at the beginning of each group session.

group for discussion: "*Superheroes have different skills and strengths. In order to solve a problem, or to save the world, they need to use all of their different skills and work together as a team. How do they decide upon their roles to work as an effective group? How do they maintain a positive relationship with one another?*"

Group members are then instructed to choose a sand tray miniature of a superhero of their choice. As they are choosing their miniature, they should think about what they believe to be the superhero's number one signature strength. They should also be prepared to share an example of a time they have demonstrated that very same strength. For example, if an individual chooses the superhero Black Panther, they may identify Black Panther's signature strength as leadership. The individual would then discuss how they have utilized that strength, perhaps while playing sports or when working on a group assignment in school. As each group member shares their superhero and strength, they place the miniature into the tray.

The intervention ends with the group members working together to create a superhero mantra and a symbol to represent their group (a large cardboard cutout of a shield has been utilized with success by allowing each group member to contribute to the shield). At the conclusion of this activity, group members may take some time to participate in "strengths-spotting". Strengths-spotting involves recognizing and labeling strengths in others (Niemiec, 2017). Group members may share which strengths they observed in others during the activity. This intervention reinforces to the group that each member possesses strengths of a superhero and that everyone's strengths should be celebrated and valued.

Our Battle Scars: Transforming Wounds into Gold

Superheroes, like Wolverine, present an undeniable metaphor for resilience in that they have shown us time and time again, their ability to get back up after being knocked down. Metaphors from comic books, video games, and anime can be the guide to therapeutic change. This intervention utilizes the Japanese art form of Kintsugi as a visual representation of recovery and can be a way to reframe hardships. The word *Kintsugi* comes from the Japanese word Kin (golden) and tsugi (joining), which translates to "golden joinery". It involves repairing a broken object with lacquer and highlighting the cracks with real gold powder (Carnazzi, 2020). The gold is an opportunity to highlight the journey, not hide it. This embraces the idea that healing happens in connection, not perfection. Essentially, this process is analogous to the hard work our clients do in their trauma healing journey.

The anime *Land of the Lustrous* portrays a world that is constantly in a break and repair cycle. It follows the story of humanoid creatures called the Lustrous, who are the embodiment of gemstones (Kyogoku, 2017). The anime symbolizes the spirit of Kintsugi in that it shows the heroes embracing their wounds instead of hiding them. Each episode provides a storyline rich in therapeutic metaphors centered on the idea that one must pick up the remains one piece at a time and weave them back together to create something stronger. Even as fragile gems, we see these characters become malleable and adapt to change. Their individuality and personal struggles are illuminated, not hidden, in their cracks and breaks. Their cracks become both a celebration of what they once were, and what they now are. In a group setting, the facilitator may play clips from the anime and pause for discussion. Group members can then be guided in creating their own artwork demonstrating their own "cracks and breaks", as well as the resiliency of their healing journey. Broken pottery pieces, toys, LEGO® bricks, and even blank puzzle pieces may be used, with the client bonding the pieces together with gold glitter glue. Clear glue may also be used and painted gold afterwards as well. Group members are instructed to write their strengths on each piece of broken pottery or blank puzzle piece. There is something inherently powerful in the process of repairing a broken item and being reminded, piece by piece, that when celebrating imperfections and repairing the things that have broken, individuals can create something far more beautiful and resilient than ever before.

Foe to Friend: Be Kind to Yourself

The mind of an adolescent is often full of the storyline that they are not good enough. Their self-critical thoughts can prove to be the ultimate villain in their own narratives. Self-compassion can be one of the most valuable superpowers an individual can possess. We can think of self-compassion as our magical cloak that embraces us with warm acceptance and kindness. It can show us that love is a far more effective motivator than fear. Compassion for others and self-acceptance are major themes in the *Ms. Marvel* comic books featuring Kamala Khan. Kamala is a Muslim, Pakistani-American teenage superhero with shapeshifting abilities. She attempts to juggle the complexities of super heroism and high school and all that it entails (self-image, bullies, relationships). In the comic book *Ms. Marvel #2* (Wilson, 2014), Kamala's first attempt into shapeshifting leads her to become a blonde-haired, blue-eyed version of the previous Ms. Marvel, Carol Danvers. Kamala chooses this form to better fit the stereotypical image of a superhero. She later finds that this does not make her happy and she makes the decision to be her authentic self. As Kamala says, "Being someone else isn't liberating. It's exhausting" (Wilson, 2014, p. 14). By choosing not to conform and accepting herself as she is, she practices self-kindness. We also see many examples of Kamala showing compassion for others by standing up for those who have been treated unjustly. The breadth of storylines available in comic books like *Ms. Marvel* can lead to a rich discussion on social skills, cognitive distortions, problem solving skills, and the importance of teamwork.

We can use the landscape of a comic book or the scene of a film or television show to explore characters' emotional arcs and personal struggles. These powerful storylines can serve as a reminder that everyone, even superheroes, have moments of inadequacy, shame, sadness, anger, and fear. Knowing that our favorite hero struggles and has moments where they must acknowledge their humanity can make us feel less alone. We can use the example above in which Kamala Khan struggles between the rift of her identities, to explore what it means to suffer and struggle.

Group members can also be directed to write a letter to a superhero in need. Directions for this activity can be given as follows: "*Think about a time when a close friend has felt really bad about him or herself or is really struggling in some way. How did you respond? Please write a letter to this superhero as if you were their best friend. What would you say to them?*" After the group has worked to create a letter together, each member then writes a new version of the letter by replacing the superhero's name with their own name. After each member has read their letter aloud, the group can then discuss whether they noticed any difference in turning that compassion toward themselves. Each group member then expands that compassion toward the entire group by offering kind words to one another. Several self-compassion interventions, including letter writing and loving-kindness exercises can be found on the website, https://self-compassion.org/. Like Ms. Marvel, adolescents often feel like outsiders peering in. The superpower of self-compassion can light the path to acceptance of self and others, allowing us to take on any new superhero adventures that lie ahead.

Group Example

This is a case example of using the *Caped Crusaders* program to facilitate group therapy for four male adolescents struggling with low self-esteem. Over the years, this author has utilized video games in play therapy groups to help increase opportunities for group connection and engagement. Video games have led to some of the most meaningful group experiences in the *Caped Crusaders* program by providing group members an opportunity for social connection and the ability to engage in self-discovery. Minecraft™ is a favorite game used in the group therapy sessions. Adolescents are familiar with the game; it is easy to use and accessible. Minecraft™ is an immersive video game that can be equated to a virtual playground where anything can be built and created. During the initial group session, the participants were given the directive, "Build Your Superhero Headquarters" in Minecraft.™ Group members are prompted to build their superhero headquarters together and to represent at least one of their signature strengths within the structure. This fun, creative, and interactive intervention can also be implemented in the sand tray.

Following the building of their headquarters, group members were taught about signature strengths and exploring what their personal signature strengths may be. They opted to each choose a different strength and build their own section of the building. Each room of the building would serve a unique purpose for their superhero team.

Strength spotting requires a careful observation of others and seeing strengths in action. Group members were encouraged to name the strengths they saw in use during the building process. Below is a list of each group member's strengths and the structures they built to represent those strengths (The *Caped Crusaders* uses the VIA Classification as a common language for strengths. The free VIA survey and list of character strengths can be found at www.viacharacter.org.)

Hassan: Leadership/Mission Control
Jamal: Love/Med Bay
Vivek: Humor/Recreation Center
Andrew: Appreciation of Beauty and Excellence/Hydroponics Lab.

After the building process concluded, group members gave a tour of their structures and discussed how each space represented their chosen signature strength. The level of ingenuity as each structure illuminated their strengths and came together to create a technologically advanced and versatile superhero lair. When asked to share which strengths were observed, Vivek reported that he noticed a lot of teamwork as others readily shared their resources and materials. Andrew noted that Jamal, whose top strength is love, took the initiative to build a bridge to connect all the buildings to make one cohesive unit. All group members shared that it was easier for them to observe strengths in others than in themselves and expressed feeling appreciated and valued during the building process. Group members agreed that the character strengths that were higher on their strengths list were more frequently utilized during the activity. The group facilitator observed expressions of engagement and excitement (enthusiasm in tone of voice and several virtual high fives) as group members recognized the positive qualities in one another. One of the most poignant discussions revolved around the strength of perspective. Hassan shared that he was better able to understand the layout and design of the structure when flying above the buildings. This led to a rich discussion on how the strength of perspective can be used to help manage personal and social challenges in everyday life.

By integrating clients' interests (video games) and pairing it with a strengths-spotting exercise, group members were provided a space to express themselves, be validated and recognized by others, and feel a sense of belonging and community.

Conclusion

Research on post-traumatic growth (PTG) suggests that there is an immense human capacity for growth and resilience after trauma and adversity. Some key predictors of positive psychological change include positive relationships, identifying and applying personal strengths, cognitive reframing, meaning making, and exercising a compassionate stance towards ourselves and others. Examples of PTG are woven into the very fabric of superhero stories. The

Caped Crusaders incorporates these inspiring and transformative stories into evidence-based therapies to help group members gain insight into their thoughts, feelings, and behaviors. Through the use of metaphors, expressive arts, self-compassion, and mindfulness practices, group members enhance their perspective about the ways they relate to their inner world and how this becomes reflected in their relationships with others. Superheroes can serve as a powerful reminder that trauma and tragedy are not the defining factor in a hero's life. Young people may struggle with understanding their emotional experiences. It can be through these powerful connections with fictional heroes, that individuals can survive, thrive, and find meaning in painful experiences. From Yoda's teachings to Batman's immense bravery, we learn that one does not need unnatural abilities to face our villains. Through the power of relationships, cultivating our strengths, and self-compassion, can we become masters of our own destiny. So, grab your capes or your lightsabers, and remember – you are a beacon of courage, a force to be reckoned with; a superhero.

References

Ansari, S. & Scott, C. M. (2019). Flourishing after the origin story: Using positive psychology to explore well-being in superheroes and supervillains. In L. C. Rubin (Ed.), *Using superheroes and villains in counseling and play therapy* (pp. 9–28). Routledge.

Bluth, K. (2017). *The self-compassion workbook for teens: Mindfulness and compassion skills to overcome self-criticism and embrace who you are.* New Harbinger Publications.

Bluth, K. & Eisenlohr-Moul, T. A. (2017). Response to a mindful self-compassion intervention in teens: A within-person association of mindfulness, self-compassion, and emotional well-being outcomes. *Journal of Adolescence*, 57, 108–118. doi:10.1016/j.adolescence.2017.04.001.

Bluth, K., Gaylord, S. A., Campo, R. A., Mullarkey, M. C., & Hobbs, L. (2015). Making friends with yourself: A mixed methods pilot study of a mindful self-compassion program for adolescents. *Mindfulness*, 7(2), 479–492. doi:10.1007/s12671-015-0476-6.

Cardona, J. (2020). *The geek therapy playbook: How to use comics, games, and movies to understand each other, and ourselves. Geek Therapy Books.* Kindle Edition.

Carnazzi, S. (2020, June 15). *Kintsugi: The art of precious scars.* LifeGate. https://www.lifegate.com/kintsugi.

Ciarrochi, J., Kashdan, T. B., & Harris, R. (2013). The foundations of flourishing. In T. B. Kashdan & J. Ciarrochi (Eds.), *Mindfulness, acceptance, and positive psychology* (pp. 1–29). Context Press.

Gander, F., Proyer, R. T., Ruch, W., & Wyss, T. (2012). Strength-based positive interventions: Further evidence for their potential in enhancing well-being and alleviating depression. *Journal of Happiness Studies*, 14(4), 1241–1259. doi:10.1007/s10902-012-9380-0.

Germer, C. & Barnhofer, T. (2017). Mindfulness and compassion: Similarities and differences. In P. Gilbert (Ed.), *Compassion: Concepts, research and applications* (1st ed., pp. 69–86). Routledge.

Germer, C. K. & Neff, K. (2015). Cultivating self-compassion in trauma survivors. In V. M. Follette, J. Briere, D. Rozelle, J. W. Hopper, & D. I. Rome (Eds.), *Mindfulness-oriented interventions for trauma: Integrating contemplative practices* (1st ed., pp. 43–58). The Guilford Press.

Hayes, S. C., Strosahl, K., & Wilson, K. G. (1999). *Acceptance and commitment therapy: An experiential approach to behavior change.* Guilford Press.

Hsu, C.-T., Conrad, M., & Jacobs, A. M. (2014). Fiction feelings in Harry Potter. *NeuroReport*, 25(17), 1356–1361. doi:10.1097/wnr.0000000000000272.

Kabat-Zinn, J. (2009). *Wherever you go, there you are: Mindfulness meditation in everyday life* (10th ed.). Hachette Books.

Kyogoku, T. (Director). (2017). *Land of the Lustrous* [Animated television series]. Japan: Orange.

Lucas, G. (Director). (1999). *Star Wars: Episode I – The Phantom Menace* [Motion picture]. United States: 20th Century Fox.

MacConville, R. (2012). *Building happiness, resilience and motivation in adolescents: A positive psychology curriculum for well-being.* Jessica Kingsley Publishers.

Neff, K. (2011). *Self-compassion: The proven power of being kind to yourself.* William Morrow Paperbacks.

Neff, K. D. & McGehee, P. (2010). Self-compassion and psychological resilience among adolescents and young adults. *Self and Identity*, 9(3), 225–240. doi:10.1080/15298860902979307.

Niemiec, R. (2017). *Character strengths interventions: A field guide for practitioners.* Hogrefe Publishing.

Peterson, C. & Seligman, M. (2004). *Character strengths and virtues: A handbook and classification* (1st ed.). American Psychological Association / Oxford University Press.

Prati, G. & Pietrantoni, L. (2009). Optimism, social support, and coping strategies as factors contributing to posttraumatic growth: A meta-analysis. *Journal of Loss and Trauma*, 14(5), 364–388. doi:10.1080/15325020902724271.

Southwick, S. M., Bonanno, G. A., Masten, A. S., Panter-Brick, C., & Yehuda, R. (2014). Resilience definitions, theory, and challenges: Interdisciplinary perspectives. *European Journal of Psychotraumatology*, 5(1), 25338. doi:10.3402/ejpt.v5.25338.

Tedeschi, R. G., Shakespeare-Finch, J., Taku, K., & Calhoun, L. G. (2018). *Posttraumatic growth: Theory, research, and applications.* Routledge.

Vezzali, L., Stathi, S., Giovannini, D., Capozza, D., & Trifiletti, E. (2014). The greatest magic of Harry Potter: Reducing prejudice. *Journal of Applied Social Psychology*, 45(2), 105–121. doi:10.1111/jasp.12279.

Wilson, G. W. (2014). *Ms. Marvel #2* (p. 14). Marvel.

4 AutPlay® Therapy Play Groups for High Needs Autistic Children

Tracy Turner-Bumberry and Robert Jason Grant

Special note: the authors are switching between the terms "children/people/ individuals with autism" and "autistics" to fully respect those who identify with either term.

Social connection and relationships are an aspect of wellness which help individuals feel happy, healthy, and whole. Children desire social relationships and can often be seen in various settings playing games and having fun with their peers. Although it is equally healthy for children to learn to be comfortable being alone, playing in a group is vital for developing appropriate social/ relational skills and confidence. There is often a misinterpretation that autistic children prefer to be alone. Those with autism typically want to have meaningful social relationships, but social situations can be difficult and anxiety provoking, and they may choose instead to withdraw (Grant, 2018). Autistic children who have a greater degree of social and engagement deficits often want to form social connection as well, but typically require additional guidance from their caregivers, teachers, and therapists.

Children with autism who are considered to be more severely impaired are challenged not only with social, relational, and play ability, but often struggle with basic interaction and engagement ability. These children would be classified by the American Psychiatric Association's *Diagnostic and Statistical Manual* (DSM) (2013) as a level three – requiring very substantial support; having severe deficits in verbal and nonverbal social communication skills and great distress/difficulty changing actions or focus. It's important for therapists to remember that those with autism who are more severely impaired (high needs) still crave social relationships and connection the same as neurotypical children, but they will need guidance and tools to learn how to navigate through social processes. As challenges are addressed, it is critical to honor the unique types of friendships autistic children may choose to have and celebrate what children with autism bring to social relationships. Providing skill development guidance to autistic children does not mean trying to change their personalities to fit a neurotypical model, rather, teaching these important skills helps them to build the confidence and capabilities needed to make and keep relationships.

DOI: 10.4324/9781003094531-4

In the late 1990s, Judy Singer, a sociologist diagnosed with autism, came up with a word to describe conditions such as autism, this word was "*neurodiversity*" (Grant, 2021). Her objective was to shift the focus of discourse about ways of thinking and learning away from the usual litany of deficits, disorders, and impairments. Neurodiversity means looking at a condition such as autism as a part of who the person is and to take away the autism is to take away the person. As such, neurodiversity activists reject the idea that autism should be cured, advocating instead for celebrating autistic forms of communication and self-expression, and for promoting support systems that allow people with autism to live as someone with autism (Disabled World, 2020).

The challenge for the group therapist working with this population is to provide an atmosphere that helps children improve their happiness and success while respecting their neurodiversity. This requires a mindfulness on the part of the therapist to carefully assess needs versus trying to make children with autism look neurotypical. This process is critical for those with autism who may need assistance with social constructs that do not manifest naturally. Starting early in life, most social and relational skills develop without formal instruction in neurotypical individuals. Neurotypical children acquire social and relational ability as part of their daily experiences and developmental growth. As such, they rarely need direct instruction on relational and social navigation, rather, they learn these valuable skills through observation, practice, and repetition. A play therapy group approach provides the opportunity to help those severely impaired by autism to gain social/relational abilities without interjecting ableism into the therapeutic process.

Overview and Research

Autistic children may fail to demonstrate the skills required to successfully initiate and sustain interactions. Some commonly observed challenges or differences include a lack of social initiations and responses, interactive play, social speech, empathy, and joint attention (Macpherson, Charlop, & Miltenberger, 2014). Challenges in social and communication skills are primary characteristics of individuals with autism (Baron-Cohen, 2004). Autistic children (especially those with higher needs) may not frequently respond to peers or adults, initiate interactions, or speak spontaneously (Ganz & Flores, 2008). The resulting lack of social engagement is believed to negatively impact the development of communicative, academic, adaptive, and relational skills. Autism is a huge spectrum, and no two autistic people are the same. Autism comes with a variety of presentations in cognitive functioning and intelligence. Often those who are nonverbal or present with a lower IQ are often perceived as being unintelligent while the opposite may be the case. Typically, even when an autistic person cannot speak or has limited engagement ability, they will have other skills in which they are fluent such as math, art, music, etc. (Vormer, 2018). These skills and interests can often be harnessed to help improve relational ability.

Cognitive functioning is an important predictor of response to any group intervention and functional outcomes in individuals with autism (Hinnebusch et al., 2017; Rivard et al., 2015). In particular, children with autism and comorbid cognitive delays appear to make limited developmental progress over time and show greater challenges in adaptive functioning, social skills, and disruptive behavior even with intensive intervention, perhaps suggesting that those who are more severely impaired may struggle to respond to traditional autism specific intervention services (Miller, Burke, Robins, & Fein, 2018).

Studies have shown that compared to neurotypical children, those with autism are less involved in group play and social activities, engage in fewer appropriate play behaviors and inconsistently respond to peers when the peers initiate play with them (Chester, Richdale, & McGillivray, 2019). What seems to be logical and "normal" play behavior to neurotypical children may seem odd, nonsensical, or irrelevant to those with autism. Children with autism may play in a way that seems confusing to neurotypical children which hinders connection and causes even more isolation and lack of social relationships to be formed.

Jamison and Schuttler (2017) proposed that social and engagement ability involves a complex set of skills that evolves over the course of human development. Autistic children often find the social functioning world confusing, frustrating, and even scary. There is a great need for them to develop the ability to categorize and understand social systems in a way that makes sense and enables them to navigate the social situations in which they are asked to participate. For autistic children to accomplish the social related goals and experiences that are important to them, they must find meaning in social functioning. Koenig (2012) proposed that social competency does not develop in isolation from cognitive, emotional, and behavioral development. There is a continual interplay among these domains and competencies. When planning or implementing social skill interventions, the whole child must be considered, otherwise the interventions may not be fully effective and may result in gaps in the child's understanding and execution of newly learned skills.

Chester, Richdale, and McGillivray (2019) identified that social and play skills training groups and programs have emerged as a popular intervention for children with autism. They are considered an evidence-based practice, endorsed as such by both the National Professional Development Center on Autism and the National Standards Project in the United States. Research has further supported peer groups as being effective in autistic children gaining social and engagement ability (Grant, 2017; Koening, 2012; Ware, Ohrt, & Swank, 2012). AutPlay® Therapy Play Groups provide a peer atmosphere which utilizes play to help autistic children with high needs gain valuable social and relational skills while honoring each group member's unique personality and strengths. This model is used with autistic children who have greater challenges in the areas of social, engagement, and connection development.

AutPlay® Therapy Play Groups is a relational-based approach which integrates elements of other established autism approaches and can easily be combined with additional autism interventions (Grant & Turner-Bumberry, 2020). The child and parent participate in these groups together and specific focus is given to developing therapeutic relationships as well as building upon the child's natural interests. The uniqueness of each child is not merely tolerated, but completely respected and valued. Social and relational skill development is built upon each group member's strengths and social skill engagements are designed to provide meaning for each child. AutPlay® Therapy Play Groups allow children who may have solely been playing alone to discover and benefit from the joys of meaningful connection and relationship.

AutPlay® Therapy Play Groups for Children with High Needs

AutPlay® Therapy Play Groups are based on the Follow Me Approach (FMA) in AutPlay® Therapy (Grant & Turner-Bumberry, 2020). The FMA is used with children who have difficulty focusing on and being able to participate in directive play therapy interventions, as well as children too young to participate in directive interventions. These children typically do not have engagement and attunement ability and lack the ability to engage with another person. These children may be nonverbal or limited in verbal ability and may be impaired cognitively. While the FMA approach is often used with younger children, AutPlay® Therapy Play Groups can also apply to older children or adolescents. The FMA focuses on relationship development, skill development, and a progression from a child's inability to focus and engage with others to participating fully in co-experienced play interventions with professionals and parents (Grant, 2017).

In FMA, the professional and child participate in a typical play therapy room environment. The child is given no directive instructions from the professional other than a structuring statement to begin the session such as "This is the playroom, and you can play with anything you want and I will be in here with you." The professional follows the child's lead, moving with the child around the playroom and trying to engage with the child in whatever activity or toy they are playing with. The professional lets the child lead but always tries to get involved in what the child is doing. The professional transitions as the child transitions and is continuously looking for opportunities to connect with the child through joint attention, verbalizations, reciprocal play, or any other play and social goals that are being targeted.

Grant and Turner-Bumberry (2020) proposed that throughout the FMA session, the professional is using reflecting and tracking statements and being mindful of the child's comfort level. In the FMA, it is important to not only share physical space with the child, but also share attention, emotion, and understanding with the child. In AutPlay® Therapy Play Groups the therapist is active in implementing the FMA principles as well as other group dynamics. Hull (2014) noted that the role of the therapist in autism groups provides a model for group members in which they can observe the behavior of the therapist as a form of learning and incorporating what they need to see in their life. Sweeney, Baggerly, and Ray (2014) furthered that the group play therapist has a crucial role in the functioning and success of the group process. There is an importance in modeling what is expected and exhibiting a belief in the process, and communication of this belief to group members. In AutPlay® Therapy Play Groups, the professional models, communicates, organizes, and facilitates the play group process. The professional is both a participant and encourager for the children and the parents. Often, the professional serves as a role model and a teacher.

Parent training and participation has been shown to be an effective and evidence-based practice when working with children with autism (Booth & Jernberg, 2010; Dempsey, Kelly-Vance, & Ryalls, 2013; Grant, 2017; Van-Fleet, 2014). In the FMA, parents work with the professional in learning how to have special play times at home with their child. Parents are taught how to have FMA play times at home with their child and thus become co-change agents in helping their child develop skills. Autistic children who have higher needs often require more directive guidance to improve challenges that are impeding their quality of life. Using the FMA framework, parents participate fully in AutPlay® Therapy Play Groups. Parents participate with their child and other parents/children during in-clinic group meetings as well as host a play time meeting outside of the clinic to help further the acquisition of social play gains. This process is fully explained to parents during the initial consultation about the play group.

AutPlay® Therapy Play Groups follow an organizational format (highlighted in Table 4.1) and are designed for three general types of children affected by autism:

1   Preschool-aged autistic children: regardless of need level, these young children often find the natural medium of play beneficial in gaining social and relational comfort and skill development.
2   Autistic children with more severely impaired social, relational, and engagement skills: these children typically require a less directive structure and the inclusion of their parents to participate and accept challenge in developing attunement and interactive ability.
3   Autistic children with high levels of resistance towards therapeutic interventions: these children may have higher social and interactive

Table 4.1 Group Establishment Steps

Step 1	*The role of the professional/therapist*
Step 2	The structure of the group
Step 3	Generating interest in the group
Step 4	Organization of the group
Step 5	Screening/assessing potential participants
Step 6	Establishing the group size (how many participants)
Step 7	The length of the group meetings (1 hour, longer, or shorter)
Step 8	The number of group meetings (10 or a different amount)
Step 9	Group meeting location
Step 10	Unexpected behavior plan

skills but may value control and be resistant towards directive activities. A less directive play approach may lead to more participation and therapeutic progress.

AutPlay® Therapy Play Groups Session Example

Special note: This example mentions specific forms used in AutPlay® Therapy Play Groups. All of these forms, as well as all group session protocols can be found in the book, *AutPlay® Therapy Play and Social Skills Groups: A 10-Session Model* (Grant & Turner-Bumberry, 2020).

Length of the Group Session

Based on a fifty-minute group session.

About This Week's Group

The therapist should take note of any specific information they want to cover or address in this group session. The therapist should review and prep for the session time. Are there any specific toys or materials that need to be highlighted? Does the room need any adjustments? Is the Session Overview Form (described later in this chapter) completed and ready to give to parents? During the first session the children will follow the professional out of the waiting room and into the playroom. Parents will remain in the waiting room until they join the group with about twenty minutes left.

The Table

This is typically a literal table (usually a small child's table with chairs) but could also be a space on the floor. This is for displaying selected toys or materials designed to promote social interaction. In AutPlay® Therapy Play Groups the children are free to roam the playroom or play space and play with anything they want. There may also be times when the therapist may want to place specific toys or materials on the "Table" to promote children playing together. Utilizing the "Table" concept is optional and may not be done in each session but should be considered as another tool to help promote social play.

Structuring Statement

Once the therapist has greeted everyone in the waiting room and all the children are in the playroom, the therapist will make a simple structuring statement – "This is the playroom, and you can play with anything you want in here and I (we) will be in here with you." Nothing else needs to be said or explained to the children at this time.

Play and Social Time

The children will have thirty-five minutes of unstructured play time. They may play with anything they want, and the therapist will move around the playroom making tracking and reflective statements and trying to encourage interactive play with themselves and other children in the group. The therapist is not aggressive and does not force any child to interact or play with anyone else. The therapist makes consistent attempts and encourages but allows the process to develop at the child's comfort level.

Parent and Child Play Time

Parents join the group for the last twenty minutes. The therapist will get the parents from the waiting room when there is about twenty minutes left of the group time. Once the parents are in the playroom, they are given the following directive "This is your time to play and interact with your child or any other parent and child and I (we) will be in here with you." This is an opportunity for the therapist to further observe the parent/child interaction, role model play attempts with the child, and allow for more social play experiences.

Five Minute Warning

When there is around five minutes left of the group time, the therapist will make the following statement "We have five minutes left of our group time today, then it will be time to go." The therapist makes another statement when there is one minute left of group time – "We have one minute left of our group time and then it will be time to go." Parent and child are free to clean up any toys or materials or leave them. They are not asked or required to clean up after the group time is over.

Give Form to Parents

As the parent and child leave the playroom, the therapist should give each parent the Session Overview Form. This form should have been completed prior to the group meeting and provides the parents with information about what was addressed in the group meeting and information about the next weeks parent hosted play time.

Goodbye Ritual

Establishing a goodbye ritual is optional in AutPlay® Therapy Play Groups but therapists may want to consider this as an effective way to transition from play group to home. The goodbye ritual should be simple and the same one may be used to end each group meeting. This could be as simple as giving a high five to each child and parent as they leave the playroom or waving and saying "bye" to each child as they leave the room. The therapist can create their own unique goodbye ritual but should remember to keep it simple and be consistent in using the same process at the end of each group meeting.

Case Example

A group was established with five parents/children registered to attend a ten-week AutPlay® Therapy Play Group. The children ranged in age from four to five years with four of the children being male and one female. All children had been diagnosed with autism spectrum disorder and had been categorized as level three in the DSM criteria and significantly lacked attunement/engagement ability. Each parent completed the group readiness questionnaire and required forms. An explanation of the group process was provided to each parent regarding their participation in the play groups. Scheduling was also established for parent hosted play times for all group members which would take place outside of the clinic setting. The in-clinic play therapy groups consisted of one lead therapist and two assistant facilitators who were supervisees of the lead therapist. All had been trained in implementing AutPlay® Therapy Play Groups.

Sessions 1–4

Beginning sessions were highlighted by parents and children getting to know each other better and becoming more comfortable in the group process. Play interactions were more isolated between parent and child and not so involved with others in the group. The lead therapist and assistant facilitators spent a great deal of time working on engaging children with each other and teaching parents how to better engage in play attempts with their child. Tracking, reflecting, and a more naturalistic child-led process was implemented.

By the end of session 4, several parents had improved in their ability to engage in play with their child's preferred toys and activities. The parents were able to let the child lead in identifying what they enjoyed manipulating and/or playing with. One parent and child were able to play various games together in the sand tray, taking turns putting sand into a bucket and burying each other's hands. Another parent and child were able to repeatedly build towers with large cardboard bricks and knock the towers over. All parents were reporting they were experiencing play interactions with their child in ways they had not been having prior to the group involvement.

The "Table" concept item was a set of foam blocks which remained the same for sessions 1–10. The lead therapist and assistant facilitators worked to naturalistically engage each child in play and encouraging each child to interact with other children in the group. In sessions 3 and 4 two of the children in the group (with the assistance of the therapist) began to play with each other in building various items from the foam blocks on the "Table." Until session 3, these two children had predominantly played in isolation or with their parent. By the end of session 4 all the children but one had shown improvement in engaging and some reciprocal play with the therapist and assistant facilitators.

Sessions 5–6

During the working phase of the group therapy process, the facilitators observed a marked improvement in familiarity and comfort among the group participants (including both parents and children). At this point, the group had also been meeting every other week outside of the clinic for a parent hosted play time. In all, participants had experienced five to six clinic sessions and five to six parent hosted play times. The combination of the in-clinic group sessions and out of clinic parent hosted play times had greatly benefited the children and parents in forming better relationships with each other.

By the end of session 6 the therapist and assistant facilitators were able to engage with and produce meaningful reciprocal play with four of the five children. They were also able to increase the engagement, acknowledgment, and play of the children with one another. Some of the parents began to work together and play with other children. During both sessions 5 and 6 one parent had made success in interacting with another parent and child. The two children and parents were able to play a group game together using musical instruments. Another parent and child were able to share the sand tray space and join another parent and child. The children displayed the ability to engage in limited sand play together.

The parents were reporting similar results in their out of clinic play times. One report highlighted a recent play time hosted by a group parent. Several of the parents shared that their children were able to interact with each other in a finger paint play time. They would put their fingers and hands in paint and then put it on another child, touching the other child's fingers, hands, or arms. The children seemed to engage in a joint attention moment and seemed to enjoy the play time. The parents were delighted and felt encouraged to continue to provide opportunities for interactive play during the parent hosted play times.

Sessions 7–10

The final sessions of the group highlighted the children's improving skills and worked to advance the ability of each of the children in the group, giving special attention to those children who were still having challenges with engaging with others. Four of the five children were now participating with the therapist, assistant facilitators, and/or other children regularly in some form of interactive play. During sessions 7–10, the therapist focused more attention on one child who was not engaging with others to help move their progress forward. The assistant facilitators continued to engage with the other parents and children to keep advancing their newly discovered skills.

The therapist worked more exclusively with this child during the play and social time to help increase the child's play and social interaction with the therapist. Occasionally the therapist would try to include one of the other children. During the parent and child play time, the therapist worked with the parent to give them additional directives to help improve their child's engagement ability. By the end of session 10, the child was showing ability to participate in some reciprocal play with the therapist and some engagement responses with one of the other children in the group.

During the final session, as the group was ending their time together, it was decided that the group would continue to meet for five more sessions to give the children additional time to enhance their skills. It was also discussed that the parents would continue to meet for play times even after the five additional in clinic groups were finished. At the end of session 10, each child in the group had advanced in their ability to play with others, engage others in a meaningful and socially accepted manner, and improved their interaction skills. Some children showed greater advancement than others, but all the children improved from the first group session. The parents all reported positive outcomes and satisfaction with the results of the group.

Conclusion

AutPlay® Therapy Play Groups are not just about addressing social and relational skill deficits. This component is certainly present, but this alone does not provide the full description of AutPlay® Therapy Play Groups. Indeed, the heart of these groups has more to do with each participant's journey than any particular social/relational skill gain. The true definition of success in an AutPlay® Therapy Play Group is the ability of a child to find hope, confidence, and success in their abilities as a social being engaging and connecting with others.

The ability for autistic children to experience true enjoyment in a social world that has historically represented hurt and confusion is the greatest testament to the success of AutPlay® Therapy Play Groups. It represents the value and importance of facilitating these groups in communities across the world and providing more experiences for autistic children to thrive in social relationships. The more that children with autism can heal from social rejection and find a place of peace in their social world, the better off we all become. Providing safe and effective play groups is one way that this can be accomplished. Autistic children can teach us a great deal about how to appreciate and value differences and their voices must be heard. The ultimate accomplishment of AutPlay® Therapy Play Groups is helping these children feel confident and secure in social navigation and providing the platform in which they can fully display their unique and fascinating talents.

References

American Psychiatric Association. (2013). *Diagnostic and statistical manual of mental disorders* (5th ed.). Author.

Baron-Cohen, S. (2004). Autism: Research into causes and intervention. *Pediatric Rehabilitation*, 7, 73–78.

Booth, P. B. & Jernberg, A. M. (2010). *Theraplay: Helping parents and children build better relationships though attachment-based play* (3rd ed.). Jossey Bass.

Chester, M., Richdale, A. L., & McGillivray, J. (2019). Group-based social skills training with play for children on the autism spectrum. *Journal of Autism and Developmental Disorders*, 49, 2231–2242.

Dempsey, J., Kelly-Vance, L., & Ryalls, B. O. (2013). The effect of a parent training program on children's play. *International Journal of Psychology: A Biopsychosocial Approach*, 13, 117–138.

Disabled World. (2020). What is: Neurodiversity, neurodivergent, neurotypical? Retrieved from: www.disabled-world.com/disability/awareness/neurodiversity/.

Ganz, B. J. & Flores, M. M. (2008). Effects of the use of visual strategies in play groups for children with autism spectrum disorders and their peers. *Journal of Autism and Developmental Disorders*, 38, 926–940.

Grant, R. J. (2017). *Autplay therpay for children and adolescents on the Autism spectrum: A behavioral play-based approach.* (3rd ed.). Routledge.

Grant, R. J. (2018). *Understanding autism spectrum disorder: A workbook for children and teens.* AutPlay Publishing.

Grant, R. J. (2021). Foreword. In E. Gil & A. A. Drewes (Eds.), *Cultural issues in play therapy* (2nd ed.). Gilford Press.

Grant, R. J. & Turner-Bumberry, T. (2020). *AutPlay® Therapy Play and Social Skills Groups: A 10-session model.* Routledge.

Hinnebusch, A. J., Miller, L. E., & Fein, D. A. (2017). Autism spectrum disorders and low mental age: Diagnostic stability and developmental outcomes in early childhood. *Journal of Autism and Developmental Disorders, 47*, 3967–3982.

Hull, K. B. (2014). *Group therapy techniques with children, adolescents, and adults on the autism spectrum: Growth and connection for all ages.* Jason Aronson.

Jamison, T. R. & Schuttler, J. O. (2017). Overview and preliminary evidence for a social skills and self-care curriculum for adolescent females with autism: The girls night out model. *Journal of Autism Developmental Disorders, 47*, 110–125.

Koenig, K. (2012). *Practical social skills for autism spectrum disorders.* W. W. Norton.

Macpherson, K., Charlop, M. H., & Miltenberger, C. A. (2014). Using portable video modelling technology to increase the compliment behaviors of children with autism during athletic group play. *Journal of Autism Developmental Disorders, 45*, 3836–3845.

Miller, L. E., Burke, J. D., Robins, D. L., & Fein, D. A. (2018). Diagnosing autism spectrum disorder in children with low mental age. *Journal of Autism and Developmental Disorders, 49*, 1080–1095.

Rivard, M., Terroux, A., Mercier, C., & Parent-Boursier, C. (2015). Indicators of intellectual disabilities in young children with autism spectrum disorders. *Journal of Autism and Developmental Disorders, 45*, 127–137.

Sweeney, D. S., Baggerly, J. N., & Ray, D. C. (2014). *Group play therapy: A dynamic approach.* Routledge.

VanFleet, R. (2014). *Filial therapy: Strengthening the parent-child relationship* (3rd ed.). Professional Resource Press.

Vormer, R. C. (2018). Autism and intelligence. In Barboa L. B. & Bradshaw, B. B. (Eds.), *Autism what schools are missing: Voices for a new path* (pp. 122–127). Goldminds Publishing.

Ware, J. N., Ohrt, J. H., & Swank, J. M. (2012). A phenomenological exploration of children's experiences in a social skills group. *The Journal for Specialists in Group Work, 37* (2), 133–151.

5 Digital Group Play Therapy

Jessica Stone and Michael Ehrig

Digital group play therapy encompasses the same fundamentals as any other group play therapy dynamic; the medium just happens to be of a digital nature. The goal of this chapter is to introduce the reader to the power of incorporating digital tools into modern group play therapy while preserving the fundamental tenets of traditional group play therapy in both face-to-face and telehealth treatment. Since the landscape of how therapeutic services are delivered is changing quickly and drastically at the time of this manuscript, it is important to consider a variety of methods to meet the clients' needs. As this is a relatively new frontier for many, including researchers and clinicians, academic "bridges" will be made to connect multi-disciplinary concepts.

Digital Group Play Therapy Overview

Incorporating digital group play therapy (DGPT) into treatment expands the possibilities for both in-office, face-to-face sessions, and via telehealth services. Identification of appropriate hardware (devices) and software (programs) which will activate the desired therapeutic factors, along with the group dynamics and components, allows the clinician to create fun, engaging, powerful group sessions. DGPT does not ask the clinician to abandon core beliefs, rather, the core beliefs, therapeutic powers of play (Shaefer & Drewes, 2014), agents of change, and fundamental tenets of group therapy will be applied and include digital tools.

As highlighted in the text, *Digital Play Therapy* (Stone, 2020), the inclusion of digital tools into play therapy sessions is not only beneficial, it is imperative. In a field where "speaking the client's language" and "meeting the client where they are" are core beliefs, it is critical to include a client's current culture into sessions. This culture includes digital tools for many. Children born in the 2000s have been brought up as digital natives – those who have never known life without digital tools (Prensky, 2001; Stone, 2019; 2020). As a culturally sensitive field we must embrace a variety of components of our clients' culture, including interests and activities, into our work (Stone, 2020; Zimmerman, 2017).

DOI: 10.4324/9781003094531-5

Group Dynamics, Team Building, and Group Play Therapy

To build on the traditional processes of group therapy, broaden the multi-disciplinary approach, and bridge between fields, it is important to consider other arenas for their approach to group dynamics and team building. Nazzaro and Strazzabosco (2009) wrote about team building and group dynamics which apply well to the needs of play therapists. Fundamentally, both group dynamics and team building are based on the relationships within the group and apply beautifully to the use of many digital tools.

Group Dynamics

According to Nazzaro and Strazzabosco, "the term 'group dynamics' refers to the interactions between three or more people who are talking together in a group setting. Group dynamics can be studied in business settings, in volunteer settings, in classroom settings, and in social settings," (2009, p.4). Within group play therapy, dynamics occur between a) the therapist(s) and each client, b) between the clients as a group and the therapist(s), and c) between each client in a variety of constellations. A diagram would depict double-sided arrows going in all directions (see Figure 5.1). This illustrates the complexities a therapist must acknowledge and account for in group play therapy.

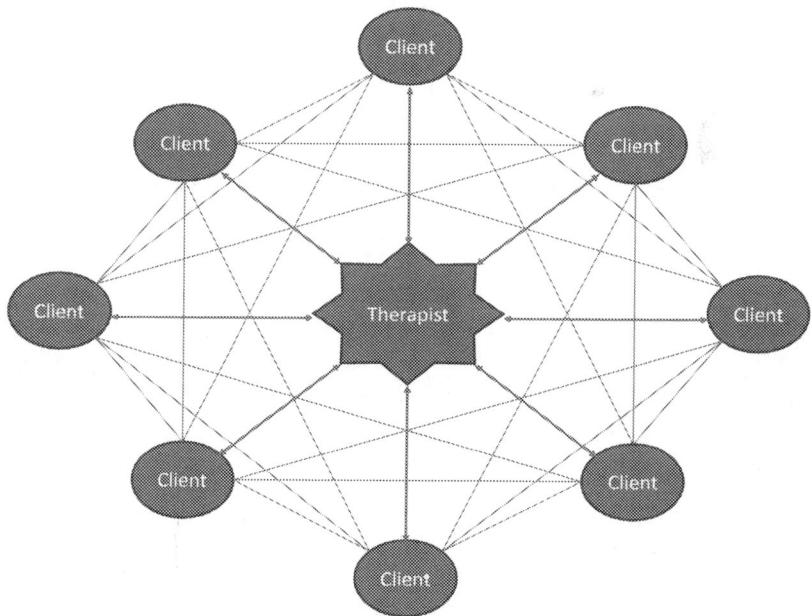

Figure 5.1 Group Play Therapy Dynamics
Source: Courtesy of Jessica Stone

Team Building

A team is a group that has a job to do, tasks to accomplish, and a goal to achieve cohesiveness (Nazzaro & Strazzabosco, 2009). Team building/work is particularly well suited to a number of digital play therapy approaches as many games include the assumption of a role within a team. Roles are influenced by everything the client brings into the group dynamic – culture, traditions, race, age, gender, etc. – along with the interplay between group members. Per Nazzaro and Strazzabosco, a team

> is a group with a common objective, whose members are very clear about working toward one purpose. It is a group whose members are interdependent. Whereas other groups may recognize the strengths of each member, team members rely on the strengths of each member to accomplish the objective. An ideal team has a number of distinct characteristics, and they fall into three areas: their feedback and communication behaviours, their behaviour and conduct courtesies, and their ways of approaching tasks and problems.
>
> (2009, p. 7)

These three areas delineated by the authors are of particular interest in digital group therapy because when clients are on a team in a game, their communication, feedback, conduct, and task management will greatly affect their role within the team, the group, and the game. These in-game interactions will elicit certain dynamics and behaviors and "an effective group is one in which those behaviours are channeled positively to move the agenda forward." (2009, p. 5). These skills apply within the digital group play and generalize to the members' day-to-day lives.

Development of Group Stages

There is a process to the development of group and team dynamics. Tailoring the therapeutic group's goals and activities according to the group developmental stages can improve the group's experience, cohesiveness, and effectiveness. Ultimately the purpose is for the therapist to recognize where the group members are in the process so the movement of the group maximizes the components of the present stage.

We can expand the traditional stages discussed in other chapters to include forming, storming, norming, performing, and transforming (please refer to Table 5.1.) (Nazzaro & Strazzabosco, 2009). To illustrate, if a group is still in the storming phase, then you cannot expect them to succeed in the performing stage; as it would be premature. Recognizing the stage the group is in as a unit, and also for each member, then tailoring the discussions and activities accordingly, will contribute to a successful group experience.

Table 5.1 Stages of Group and Team Development*

Forming	Initially the group is forming. The members may question why they are there, what the purpose of the group even is, people are often displaying their best behavior and sometimes their worst if they are dysregulated, anxious, etc., members might be more careful about what they say and do.
Storming	As the group begins to cohese and define itself, there will most likely be some disagreement and differing opinions. Additionally, group roles and positions will be assumed and defined. This is called the storming phase.
Norming	When the group develops a common goal, vision, and/or objectives, they are in the norming phase. The members are getting to know each other and how each person's strengths, abilities, knowledge, etc. will contribute to achieving the defined goals. Goals and objectives can include specific tasks to achieve but can also include getting to know each other in ways that build trust toward the performing stage. In the business world tasks may be differently oriented, but the concepts apply to therapy even if the goals differ.
Performing	When relationships and trust have been formed, the members can feel more secure in moving forward as a unit toward the defined goals. With common goals and defined roles, the members can feel less insecure about trusting the team to not hurt them in any way, particularly emotionally.
Transforming	Members are in the "zone" when the group is transforming. Trust is high, roles are secure, communication is flowing, and direction can be redefined and more quickly changed as necessary.

Note: *Adapted from Nazzaro and Strazzabosco, 2009.

Group Play Therapy

Sweeney et al., 2014, refers to group play therapy as a:

> …dynamic, interpersonal, and reciprocal relationship between two or more clients and a therapist trained in both play therapy and group therapy procedures. This involves the selection of specific expressive and projective play media, and the facilitation and development of safe relationships for clients to express and explore themselves and others (including feelings, thoughts, experiences, and behaviors). This occurs through expressive play, a natural medium of communication for children and a nonverbal means of expression for persons of all ages.
>
> (p. 3)

This play therapy specific definition includes the people involved in the group, the therapist credentials, the materials involved, the importance of the relationship, and the mechanisms of change.

When compared to individual therapy, a shift from the intra- to inter-personal focus is key in group therapy (Berg & Johnson, 1971; Berg & Landreth, 1979). This shift enables the therapist and clients to focus less on what each individual brings into the room and more on which components impact the group rules, norms, goals, and dynamics. Referring back to the stages listed above, the therapist is constantly assessing the group stage, eliciting and incorporating involvement from the members, and adjusting the group progression accordingly. In group play therapy, this also includes what play materials would be presented and why. In digital group play therapy, the goal and process are no different.

Research

Research on digital group play therapy is needed. At this time we can bridge together group therapy, play therapy group, digital therapy, and digital play therapy research and writings until specific digital group play therapy research is conducted. Further research on the use of digital tools in group play therapy will be very beneficial.

Group Play Therapy

Generally speaking, group play therapy has been found to be effective with a variety of populations, cultures, and disorders. Focusing on two international studies, effectiveness can be identified for group members both during the group sessions and in generalized future behavior shifts. These include different countries, different presenting issues, and different approaches, yet still yield within-group and outside-of-group benefits.

Morshed et al. (2019) concluded that group play therapy was effective in children who were diagnosed with Oppositional Defiant Disorder (ODD). Moreover, they found that there was not a difference in the parent or teacher reported ODD symptoms between those who participated in individual or group play therapy at the two-month mark. In other words, they compared individual and group play therapy treatment for the reduction of ODD symptoms and found 1) there was no demonstrated difference between individual and group and 2) that the benefits were retained two months later per parent and teacher reports.

Su and Tsai (2016) looked at the effect of group play therapy on new immigrants who were "exhibiting relationship difficulties". Their findings include a shift in the group member's interaction patterns from wanting to control others to listening to others. They found that the group dynamics are paramount, as one member stated "If classmates wanted me to do it, I would cooperate. If someone I don't like asked me to do something, I walked away to play with others." (p. 97). Ultimately, the children who participated in the group play therapy "experienced less interpersonal relationship difficulties, more self-control, and better confidence" (p. 100).

Digital Play Therapy

Ceranoglu (2010) posited that the therapeutic use of video games in therapy to build a relationship, evaluate cognitive processing styles, and elaborate and clarify experienced conflicts was vitally important. Granic, Lobel, and Engels (2014) explored the motivational, emotional, and social benefits of casual and serious (educational and medical uses) gaming. They state that utilizing video games in mental health treatment can "improve intervention effects across a broad spectrum of disorders" (p. 75). The Granic et al. article is rich with research findings, implications, and calls for needs to be met, including an increase in the incorporation of video games into mental health treatment.

Velez et al. (2012) conducted a study which found that cooperative game play can increase helping behaviors. Helping behaviors are key to the forming and norming stages of group development and lead the group toward the transforming stage. Horne-Moyer et al. (2014) reviewed the clinical implications of including electronic games in therapy. They found that the use of electronic/digital games in therapy in general, and group in particular

> can provide effective, efficient, and appealing interventions for a variety of clients. The psychotherapeutic use of EGE (electronic games for entertainment) as an adjunct to individual or group therapies has a long tradition that is consistent with play and group therapy in general…
>
> (p. 6)

Environment

Face-To-Face and Telehealth

Digital group play therapy can be used in both face-to-face and telehealth sessions.

In both mediums, key components to consider include: proper vetting of the digital tool – both the hardware (device) and software (program, app, etc.), discovery of what the client can access, review of one's professional board guidelines, proper discussions with the client and caregivers, and obtaining proper informed consent. The *Digital Play Therapy* book (Stone, 2020) will provide a foundation for the play therapist in these areas.

Face-to-Face

Face-to-face group digital play therapy sessions will require devices and space for all members. A typical group room would suffice unless using virtual reality, which would need a significant amount of space for each group member. Consideration for whether the therapist would provide the hardware and software, the client would provide their own, or some combination of the above would be important to establish in advance. Investing in a number of devices for face-to-face use would be beneficial.

Telehealth

The changes brought about in the spring of 2020 were swift and impactful for many play therapists and their clients. Play therapists shifted gears quickly as a profession and sessions were moved to an online platform. This swift adjustment was necessary to provide both support regarding the shocking news of the COVID-19 pandemic, the resulting changes in day-to-day life, and therapeutic continuity of care in general. It is likely these changes will have a lasting impact on how mental health treatment looks for generations. A more in-depth exploration into online group therapy can be found in Weinberg and Rolnick (2020), *Theory and Practice of Online Therapy.*

Finding multiplayer online games, apps, and programs, which allow multiple people to contribute and participate, is vital. Considerations of confidentiality, profile creation, "friending" and discoverability, and chat moderation, etc., should always be explored. The American Psychological Association (APA) (2013) established telepsychology practice guidelines, to assist those implementing this modality. Please refer to the APA guidelines for further information: https://www.apa.org/practice/guidelines/telepsychology.

Games and programs to be considered would have identifiable therapeutic powers of play (Schaefer & Drewes, 2014), components which complement the group dynamic and team stages, and are highly motivating (fun) for the clients involved. Some such games and programs include: the Virtual Sandtray App®©, Animal Crossing®, art programs such as Drawpile®, Magma®, and Aggie.io®, and a plethora of different MMO (Massively Multiplayer Online) and MOG (Multiplayer Online Game) games.

Digital Group Play Therapy Case Examples

Case Study #1 – Michal Ehrig, MA

The Nintendo WiiU is a console that allows for single or multiple users to play. A game is typically projected on a television or computer monitor. Certain games can be used in multiplayer settings so players can face each other or work together towards a common goal. The different gameplay modes are complimentary to a group setting working on social skills. The group described in this case example consisted of four boys in the 10–12-year age range who presented with social skill difficulties. The group met for 8 sessions.

Beginning Phase

In the beginning sessions clients spent time building rapport with one another by sharing what they liked about their favorite genre of games. The genres used in sessions consisted of action, fighting, strategy, and adventure. The games proposed consisted of Super Smash Bros. (fighting), Super Mario Party (turn-based board game), Hyrule Warriors (fighting/task-based game), and Super Mario 3D World (action game). The group then discussed and agreed upon group rules for the sessions which included: show respect to one another, listen without interrupting, and put effort into the gameplay. The therapist then worked with the group to agree upon the therapeutic goals, which included improved communication, taking turns, frustration tolerance, and emotional regulation.

The first game used was Super Mario 3D World which allowed the group to work together as a team. This aided the clients' rapport building and learning how to listen to each other to accomplish a task within the game. Initially, the clients struggled with being able to effectively divvy up the objectives and following the rule of letting each person take turns leading. Ultimately, the clients decided they would each have a chance to successfully lead the group on each game level before moving on to the next level. They were cognizant of the rules and remained respectful realizing they had to work together to complete the level.

The next session utilized the game Super Smash Bros. This game can be played in the form of free-for-all matches where each user is playing against all the other players, or it can be used in a team format. The first format chosen by the group was a "free-for-all", which allowed each member of the group to fight against all of the other members in the group. At the end of this match, some of the clients would brag about winning (which upset other members of the group). However, when other clients won the match they did not brag and wanted to play again. The positive response of the second group was effective modeling of maintaining respect for one another regardless of the outcome.

Middle Phase

After a few sessions, the group felt more comfortable being able to express emotions freely such as frustration, sadness, and happiness within the gameplay. At this stage, they began to play Super Mario Party. Each player rolled the dice and then moved forward on the gameboard. After each group member moved ahead, a mini game was triggered. There are three types of mini games: 1) every player for himself against the other three players, 2) two players become a team and play against the other two players, or 3) all the players work together as a team against the computer. The game itself randomly selects which type of game will be played, so the clients could not control the teams as they had in Super Smash Bros. This enhanced the clients' need to communicate with each other, to work together against either another team or the computer. This experience allowed for a more cohesive group to form, especially when they played together against the computer. By playing the different mini games and either working alone or in a group, the clients began showing flexibility in thinking and adaptive behaviors, whether they were playing alone or working together as a group.

As the group progressed, the clients discussed how the games had helped them communicate with each other, make quick decisions, and respond appropriately to changing situations. Clients were encouraging toward each other during the game play. The group learned to support each other even if one of them made a mistake.

Final Phase

In the final phase, the clients were very comfortable and easily used teamwork within the gameplay. The game Hyrule Warriors is unique because it allows players to choose individual tasks or objectives on a map, while the other players have to accomplish group objectives and tasks. The game relies heavily on the success of all the players being able to join together in order to fight the boss of the map. Additionally, this game has each player choose a specific character to play throughout an entire storyline, but the game then assigns whether the characters are going to be the "bad" ones or the "good" ones depending on the level of the game. The group members were able to see that there were different paths for different characters, although they all ended up in similar situations together.

In this game, the players would earn group currency and would need to choose which characters to upgrade using this currency. The group was able to communicate and discuss where the resources would be allocated in the game. As a result, the players decided to keep every character on the same level of strength in order to have an equally balanced team for the missions. They discussed this and came to the realization that you are only as strong as your weakest character. By ending the group with this game, it was clear that the clients had been successful in being able to meet the goals of enhancing their communication, frustration tolerance, taking turns, and emotional regulation, all while playing their favorite games and using these new successful social skills.

Case Study #2 – Jessica Stone, Ph.D., RPT-S.

Based on an eight-week session model, five clients who were poised to begin a weekly group for 10–13-year-old boys prior to the onset of

COVID-19, and the ensuing isolation, were invited to join in the remote version of the group experience. Connection during the group would be made using iPads and iPhones and virtual reality head mounted display (HMD) units, depending on the activity. The presenting concerns for the group members included: emotional expression, poor coping skills, and anger/aggression difficulties. These concerns were present in multiple environments including home, school, and in past face-to-face sessions.

Hardware and Software

iPads and iPhones – Virtual Sandtray App

Whether in person or in a telehealth session, the Virtual Sandtray App (VSA) can be used within group sessions. The main therapist's app can connect with up to eight client devices during one session for a group tray creation experience, for the group to witness one member's creation, and/ or the therapist to create a group scenario or exercise. Creating a fun, engaging VSA tray during a group meeting can contribute to group cohesion, self- and/or group- expression, rapport building, communication, and much more. The ability to connect separately to each client allows for a level of separation which can be beneficial for clients with these types of difficulties.

Virtual Reality Head Mounted Display Units – Rec Room

Each client in the group was asked prior to the remote group formation if they had access to a Virtual Reality (VR) HMD. All but one client had an HMD and this remaining client "checked" one out from the therapist. Software (games) were identified based on 1) each client having access and 2) the ability for multiplayer engagement. Rec Room was the first software identified as a common ground as it is 1) free, 2) has multiplayer engagement, and 3) can be accessed from multiple devices, including a computer or phone if any member had any technological issues along the way.

Paperwork and Discussions

Along with the traditional group paperwork and parental consent forms, both caregivers and clients were involved in verbal discussions and orientation to the use of the Virtual Sandtray App and Rec Room for the therapeutic sessions. Caregivers and clients were provided the group's therapeutic goals, fundamental rules, and the therapeutic powers of play which would be pulled for and hopefully activated during the group through the use of these programs. Caregivers were informed in writing and verbally of the risks and benefits of the use of the tools within the group session. Each family was informed that the verbal (and non-verbal) communication would be achieved and maintained through the telehealth platform and the in-program connection would be achieved separately through the appropriate device.

For the VSA, caregivers were informed they would 1) need an iPad or iPhone to be available to the client, and* 2) they would need to download the free Virtual Sandtray – Client app from the App Store. They were informed they would not need to make an account or provide any personal information whatsoever to use the VSA. The VSA is only available to the client on their device during sessions when connected to the therapist through the remote feature. (*Clients who did not have access to an iPhone or iPad were provided with an older model loaner iPhone).

Rec Room is a program which requires an account be created. Caregivers were advised to create the account with their child together so they could determine a non-identifying profile. One client already had a Rec Room account and was asked to make a second one with non-identifying information. Caregivers and clients alike were given time to ask any questions regarding the process, group, hardware, software, and more. It is critical that these front-loaded conversations occur prior to the use of such tools.

Sessions 1 and 2

Sessions 1 and 2 included the typical group cohesion discussions and connections. Each client connected to the therapist's telehealth platform via the provided secure link. Sessions were scheduled to be 90 minutes long. Group rules were discussed and agreed upon during the first session utilizing a digital whiteboard for all to see via screenshare, including specific rules for the online components of the group, i.e., muting, talking, interrupting, cameras on/off, etc. The first session concluded with each client sharing what they felt comfortable showing about their homes, their pets, their favorite things, and what they wanted to get out of the group, as well as their opinions about being involved. The second session included check-ins regarding the past week and an introduction via screenshare of the VSA to the two members who were not familiar with it. A practice run of connecting remotely with the therapist in the expanded group mode was completed. Each client was instructed to think of one fifth of the tray they would like to create next session during the week before the next meeting.

Sessions 3, 5, and 7

It was decided that the group activities would alternate weekly; one week the VSA would be used, and the next Rec Room would be used. Sessions 3, 5, and 7 would include the use of the VSA. Session 3 was a follow-up to the homework provided in session 2; to envision their contribution to the group tray 3. Each client connected to the therapist's app and was allowed to take control of the tray creation. This allowance was granted by the therapist and fully within the therapist's control to give and take it away as deemed necessary. A tray of five distinct fifths was created, one by one with each member witnessing the creation of the other members. The group tray was processed verbally, given an agreed-upon name to save it under, saved, and screenshots were taken (as was agreed upon by each member in the group unanimously – a required component).

Sessions 5 and 7 utilized two exercises: 1) *Eight Dimensions of Wellness* (Reynolds, 2017) and 2) *Things I Can and Cannot Control* ("Things I Can and Cannot Control", n.d.). In the *Eight Dimensions of Wellness* exercise, each client provided at least one model and surrounding environment which correlated with the sections: emotional, spiritual, intellectual, physical, environmental, financial, occupational, and social. Three of the group members provided a second depiction with the agreement of the remaining two members. Each identified dimension was encapsulated by a dome shield of the member's preferred color. The experience was narrated by the group, saved, and screenshots were allowed to be taken. The *Things I Can and Cannot Control* exercise included depictions of an inner area defined as the "things I can control" and the outer area of the tray as the "things I cannot control". The therapist created the areas as an inner circle dug down to the liquid layer to depict the "can control" section and the area outside the inner circle as the "cannot control". Each client was provided with the time and ability to depict their own contributions to the group tray. The tray was named, saved, and screenshots were allowed to be taken.

Sessions 4, 6, and 8

Sessions 4, 6, and 8 were held within the VR HMDs and in the Rec Room program. Each group member remained present and connected within the telehealth platform either on their phone, tablet, or computer. All discussions were held through the telehealth platform as chat features – verbal and written – may be monitored by the program and therefore are not considered private. Microphones and chat features were disabled in the VR HMDs for the group sessions. Rec Room includes numerous games and activities, and each group member chose their preferred activity over the three sessions. Team building activities were encouraged to work toward group cohesiveness. The final session included a group process discussion regarding the sessions and activities to date. Clients were asked to identify what they enjoyed and/or did not enjoy about the group, what they felt they gained, and whether or not they would like to participate in a similar group in the future. All group members wanted to join for a second 8-session group.

Conclusion

Group therapy in telehealth can initially pose a new challenge for the play therapist. Knowledge of the available digital tools, identifying the therapeutic factors, aligning the treatment goals with the available programs, and engaging the members in immersive, highly motivating activities can create a phenomenal remote telehealth group play therapy experience. Applying a solid theoretical foundation with the wide variety of available digital options leads to a solid course of treatment.

The use of such tools is relatively new to the majority of the play therapy population. Many people did not embrace the addition of such tools prior to the COVID-19 pandemic, but due to the necessity of moving to a telehealth session format, were quite surprised when they discovered how engaging and informative this type of play can be. With components one can easily identify within the therapeutic powers of play (Schaefer & Drewes, 2014), utilizing digital tools is ripe for appropriate therapeutic interactions. While there is a great need for further research, current research and direct clinical use are showing the possibilities for DGPT are virtually endless!

References

American Psychological Association. (2013). *Guidelines for the practice of telepsychology.* www.apa.org/practice/guidelines/telepsychology.

Berg, R. C. & Johnson, J. A. (1971). *Group counseling: A source book of theory and practice.* American Continental.

Berg, R. C. & Landreth, G. L. (1979). *Group counseling.* Accelerated Development.

Ceranoglu, T. A. (2010). Video games in psychotherapy. *Review of General Psychology, APA,* 14(2), 141–146.

Granic, I., Lobel, A., & Engels, R. (2014). The benefits of gaming. *American Psychologist,* 69(1), 66–78.

Horne-Moyer, H. L., Moyer, B. H., Messer, D. C., & Messer, E. S. (2014, October 14). *The Use of Electronic Games in Therapy: A Review with Clinical Implications.* www.researchgate.net/publication/266948174_The_Use_of_Electronic_Games_in_Therapy_a_Review_with_Clinical_Implications.

Morshed, N., Babamiri, M., Zemestani, M, & Alipour, N. (2019). A comparative study on the effectiveness of individual and group play therapy on symptoms of oppositional defiant disorder among children. *Korean Journal of Family Medicine,* 40, 368–372.

Nazzaro, A-M. & Strazzabosco, J. (2009, May). *Group dynamics and team building* [Conference session]. World Federation of Hemophilia. Montréal, Québec. www1.wfh.org/publication/files/pdf-1245.pdf.

Prensky, M. (2001). Digital natives digital immigrants. *On the horizon (MCB University Press)* 9(5), 1–6. www.marcprensky.com/writing/Prensky%20-%20Digital%20Natives,%20Digital%20Immigrants%20-%20Part1.pdf.

Reynolds, J. (2017). *Wellness 8.* directSMARTS.

Schaefer, C. E. & Drewes, A. (2014). *The therapeutic powers of play: 20 core agents of change* (2nd ed.). Wiley.

Stone, J. (2019). Digital Games. In Stone, J. & Schaefer, C. E. (Eds), *Game play* (3rd ed., pp. 99–115). Wiley.

Stone, J. (2020). *Digital play therapy: A clinician's guide to comfort and competence.* Routledge.

Su, S-H. & Tsai, M-H. (2016). Group play therapy with children of new immigrants in Taiwan who are exhibiting relationship difficulties. *International Journal of Play Therapy*, 25(2), 91–101.

Sweeney, D., Baggerly, J., & Ray, D. (2014). *Group play therapy: A dynamic approach*. Routledge.

"Things I can and cannot control" (n.d.).

Velez, J. A., Mahood, C., Ewoldsen, D. R., & Moyer-Guse, E. (2012, August 16). *Ingroup versus outgroup conflict in the context of violent video game play: The effect of cooperation on increased helping and decreased aggression*. https://journals.sagepub.com/doi/abs/10.1177/0093650212456202.

Weinberg, H. & Rolnick, A. (2020). *Theory and practice of online therapy*. Routledge.

Zimmerman, K. A. (2017, July 13). *What is culture?*Live science. www.livescience.com/21478-what-is-culture-definition-of-culture.html.

6 Camp Nurture

An Immersion in Key Components of TraumaPlay®

Paris Goodyear-Brown, Kate Worley, and Jennifer Rubens

Introduction to TraumaPlay®

TraumaPlay is a flexibly sequential play therapy model grounded in attachment theory and based on current understandings of the neurobiology of play, trauma, and the power of one to heal the other. This chapter describes an immersive group experience for adoptive children called Camp Nurture. The program amplifies therapeutic growth in two key areas of TraumaPlay: 1) enhancing self-regulation and 2) expanding the role of parents as partners in their child's healing. The structure of camp, the roles of camp counselors and parents during camp, and a daily schedule of group experiences will be highlighted.

The key components of the TraumaPlay model include: 1) enhancing felt safety and security; 2) augmenting coping skills; 3) soothing the physiology (enhancing self-regulation and growing parents or teachers as co-regulating partners); 4) increasing emotional literacy; 5) leveraging play-based gradual exposure; 6) addressing the thought life (helping clients to identify cognitive distortions or false attributions related to the trauma and to replace negative self-talk with positive statements, preferably through verbalization with full-body engagement) (Goodyear-Brown, 2010b); and 7) making positive meaning of the post-trauma self (Goodyear-Brown, 2019; 2010a). This model also supplies dozens of directive play therapy interventions as scaffolding to the umbrella framework of client-specific treatment goals.

Camp Nurture is an expression of TraumaPlay intended for adoptive children who have experienced multiple caregiver disruptions and who have externalizing behaviors (patterns of dysregulation) that put them at risk of having their adoptions disrupted. The week-long and multi-week-day camp formats are designed specifically to encourage a deep dive into the critical component of TraumaPlay relating to regulation: Soothing the Physiology. Broken down into treatment goals, the two main objectives of Camp Nurture are enhancing self-regulation and equipping Parents as Partners to be more effective co-regulators for their children. To this end, three features distinguish Camp Nurture from traditional day camp

DOI: 10.4324/9781003094531-6

experiences: 1) each camper has a TraumaPlay trained adult "buddy" who stays with the camper at all times, providing moment-to-moment feedback and functioning as a continuous co-regulator; 2) parents are an integral part of camp and move from involvement in parent training and support groups into active co-regulator roles over the course of camp; and 3) immersive cycles of up-and-down regulating experiences help grow the camper's skill in self-regulating as the camper's window of tolerance for distress is expanded. Campers attend a variety of groups throughout the day, including groups that offer life skills training and those that offer in-vivo practice in nurturing each other. Three areas of research provide the context for Camp Nurture's therapeutic approach (See Table 6.1).

Overview and Research

Safe Boss Buddies and Why They are Important

Camp Nurture counselors are referred to as Safe Boss Buddies (SBBs). While senior staff run the groups and are available to provide extra support when necessary, each camper has one or more individually assigned buddies. SBBs are usually therapists in training. Research supports the need for attuned, responsive caregiving for infants and young children in order for optimal regulation of abilities to develop. Psychoneurobiological mechanisms for regulation exist in the earliest attachment relationships (Schore, 2000). Tronick and Cohn (1989) view infants and caregivers as components of a dyadic co-regulation system, with each participant in this neurobiological dance influenced by the other. Termed the Mutual Regulation Model (Banella & Tronick, 2019), it has become an integral idea in what is now the field of Interpersonal Neurobiology (IPNB). Implicit forms of relational knowing, co-regulation, and eventual regulation with peers or adults stem from cycles of opening and closing circles of communication in early life (Banella et al., 2018). Combining the therapeutic powers of play (Schaefer & Drewes, 2013) with IPNB (Wheeler & Dillman Taylor, 2016) provides fun, pleasurable experiences of being connected. Research shows that consistent interactions with a guiding caregiver as children move through age-appropriate challenges helps to set up a healthy stress-response capacity, and ultimately provides the supportive context for self-regulation and executive function (Perry, 2010).

Children who begin life in institutional settings suffer from early deprivation and often have a range of developmental delays (Ainsworth, 1962; Gunnar, 2001). While these environments can vary, they are likely to have higher child to caregiver ratios, larger group sizes, and frequent turnover in caregiving staff, peer group members, or both. Adopted children may have lived in a variety of other non-parental care arrangements, including kinship care environments, placement with foster parents (sometimes further complicated by intermittent visits with biological parents), or had

Table 6.1 Areas of Research for Camp Nurture

Attachment, Co-Regulation, and the Role of Safe Boss Buddies	Adopted children often have insecure or disorganized attachment patterns when entering camp. Early attachment experiences can negatively shape the adoptive children's approach to peer relationships (Doyle & Cicchetti, 2017). Without an intensive focus on re-patterning attachment relationships, the same negative or disconnected interactions that happened with peers in prior institutional settings or foster homes might simply be repeated in the group setting. Therefore, as a precursor to successful experiences with peers, Camp Nurture prioritizes healing interactions between each camper and an assigned adult (a Safe Boss Buddy) who serves as an organizing presence (Tronick & Cohn, 1989) and is well-trained, attuned, and trauma competent.
Neuroscaffolding and Self-Regulation	Adopted children may have experienced in utero threats (such as maternal drug or alcohol use), early neglect or maltreatment, or caregiver disruptions, resulting in delays or differences in several developmental arenas. It is now well understood that experience shapes the brain; specifically, neural circuitry is use dependent (Hebb, 1949; Kay, 2009; Siegel & Bryson, 2012) and there are sequential processes to neurodevelopment (Gaskill & Perry, 2012). Leveraging this research, the camp was designed for children to gain critical experiences in a specific order repeatedly throughout the day. These playful interactions offered cyclically throughout the camp day provide a solid scaffolding that enable new neural circuitry to develop (Hong & Mason, 2016; Stewart et al., 2016). This focus on building the brain towards self-regulation is one of the goals of Trauma-Play and children benefit from the immersive experience in adult supported cycles.
The Importance of Parental Involvement	The efficacy of therapy increases for traumatized children when parents are involved in treatment (Carr, 2008). Parents are required to participate in Camp Nurture and attend their own psychoeducation and support groups throughout the camp day. As a result of their participation, parents can make significant paradigm shifts (Goodyear-Brown, 2021) that will support their children well beyond the camp experience by providing skill sets specific to caring for the challenging child.

multiple foster care placements. More frequent caregiver disruptions are correlated with higher numbers of externalizing or internalizing problems by age twelve (Almas et al., 2020).

Adopted children who are referred to Camp Nurture usually exhibit aggressive or impulsive behaviors and are often dysregulated, both at home and school. These children need to have their brains and bodies retrained in the context of interpersonal relationships that also offer attunement and positive emotion (Gaskill & Perry, 2017). The SBB provides the ongoing interpersonal relationship; sticking together with their camper (within three feet) at all times.

Their primary job is to attune to the child in their care to provide co-regulation as needed. SBBs close proximity to their campers (within three feet) provides a relationship that is attuned to the child's stress response system as they move through cycles of excitation and soothing.

These helpers are trained to embody the three roles of TraumaPlay trained caregivers: Safe Boss, Nurturer, and Storykeeper (Goodyear-Brown, 2021). The SBBs build trust with their campers and establish Safe Boss status by moving between *secure base* behaviors (supporting the camper's exploration while watching over their camper, delighting in them, and helping them when needed) and *safe haven* behaviors (welcoming them back in their distress) (Powell et al., 2013). SBBs become Nurturers as they offer food, drink, nurturing touch, novel play experiences, and attune to their camper's needs. Finally, SBBs become Storykeepers for their camper by meeting with the parents; understanding the trauma history of the child and how their current problematic behaviors may be the outgrowth of early trauma experiences or maladaptive coping that was useful in helping them survive prior to adoption. Campers often share pieces of their trauma story with their SBB over the course of camp, and part of their training involves stretching their capacity for holding hard stories and validating big feelings.

The Role of Parents as Partners in Camp Nurture

As noted earlier, parents are required to fully participate in Camp Nurture. Adopted children often have more than one adverse childhood experience (ACE) (Anthony et al., 2019). Having a trusted adult in childhood significantly decreases the risk of negative mental health outcomes for children who experience early adversity (Bellis et al., 2017). However, adoptive and foster parents may themselves have been shaped by early adversity (Adkins et al., 2020), may have differences in reflective capacity, or may have been trained in traditional parenting approaches (those that assume a secure attachment) that are not optimal for children with attachment wounds. These parents benefit from a broad landscape of psychoeducation, including a deeper understanding of bottom-up brain development (the need to provide regulation-based experiences, connecting with the feeling brain before attempting to reason with the thinking brain (Siegel & Bryson, 2012), the caregiving roles of healthy attachment figures (Hoffman et al., 2017), the sensory regulation needs of neglected or maltreated children (Kranowitz, 1998), how their own attachment history may influence their current parenting practices (Siegel & Hartzell, 2013), and how to avoid arming the fear-based brain). The format of Camp Nurture ensures that parents are able to participate in psychoeducational group experiences while their adoptive child is growing therapeutically in the care of trauma-competent SBBs.

Parents also benefit from the reminder that they are not alone. Parents of adoptive children, especially those with externalizing behaviors, can feel very isolated and unsupported (McKirdy et al., 2019). Many adoptive parents enter their new roles with the minimal training provided by the adoption agency and feel they would benefit from additional training (Barnett et al., 2018). At Camp Nurture, support groups focus on normalizing their shared experiences, reminding them that they are not alone, and helping to build a sense of community that can last far beyond the closing ceremonies of camp. Adopted children, especially when easily dysregulated, do not handle transitions easily which makes it difficult for parents to get child care assistance; leaving children with an untrained babysitter, for example, can be untenable. The Camp Nurture combination of psychoeducational groups and support groups focuses on creating paradigm shifts, re-opening each parent's compassion well, enhancing skill acquisition, and creating safe environments where parents can engage in Reflective Attachment Work (reflecting on their own early attachment relationships, see Goodyear-Brown, 2021) to better prepare them to be attuned, regulated adults, available for helping co-regulate their children. Parents slowly enter the camp experience, starting in a cheerleading capacity, delighting in their children's big body achievements (e.g., clapping for them when they climb to the top of the rope ladder during Big Body Movement time where children get the sensory break time needed to help with regulation). Parents next observe the buddies as they co-regulate and connect with the camper in their care; then, slowly, they begin to take risks of their own, implementing new Safe Boss Behaviors with their children while being fully supported by the buddies. Parents can ask clarifying questions, engage in facilitated moments of repair, process parental emotions, and help other parents stretch their reflective capacities and their windows of tolerance for distress.

Soothing the Physiology: Expanding the Window of Tolerance

Neglect, maltreatment, and chronic trauma can negatively impact the child's window of tolerance (Siegel, 2010), creating states of hypo-arousal and hyperarousal (Ogden et al., 2006). Adoptive children who struggle with dysregulation are easily kicked out of their optimal arousal zone. Children who did not have a supportive attachment figure to help mitigate stress for them early in life tend to move outside their optimal arousal window much more frequently than children who had thousands of repetitions of nurturing care early in life. At Camp Nurture, the co-regulation strategies codified in the acronym SOOTHE are taught to both SBBs and to the parenting groups. These strategies include Soft tone of voice and face, Organize, Offer, Touch or physical proximity, Hearing the underlying anxiety, and End and let go (see Goodyear-Brown, 2021 for a more extensive treatment of these concepts).

The creation of felt safety in relationship to a SBB sets the stage for the child to use the Buddy as a co-regulator while working towards self-regulation. The processes of up-regulating (having a dance party or moving through our big body movement circuit) and downregulating (snuggling with a buddy, engaging in yoga exercises with their buddies, engaging in deep breathing or resting under a weighted blanket while listening to a story) encourage the expansion of the window of tolerance (Siegel, 2010).

When a child is engaging in disruptive behavior, SBBs are encouraged to view the behavior as a signal that something is needed (Goodyear-Brown, 2021). Behavior is viewed through the lens of triune brain development (MacLean, 1990). The reptilian brain stem, the lowest brain region and the first to begin developing in utero, is responsible for heart rate, respiration, body temperature, and bodily functions driven by the autonomic nervous system. The healthy functioning of the hypothalamic-pituitary-adrenal (HPA) axis can be compromised by early adverse care experiences (Koss et al., 2016). Early deprivation and neglect may become biologically embedded in the stress response system of adopted children (Reilly & Gunnar, 2019). Post-institutional adoptions have significant differences in sensory integration including deficits in several sensory processing domains (touch, movement-avoids, movement-seeks, vision, and audition) as well as behavioral domains (activity level, organization, and social emotional) (Cermak & Daunhauer, 1997). Camp Nurture staff are trained to ask these questions: Has the camper had the nourishment they need as many adopted children benefit from a protein rich snack every couple of hours (Purvis et al., 2007)?, Have they had enough hydration?, Are they getting optimal amounts of sensory input? Adopted children often have increased sensory seeking behavior, increased sensory defensiveness, or a combination of both (Wilbarger et al., 2010) and may need their buddies to offer them a different physical activity. Once they have established that regulation of the brain stem is supported, they move to co-regulating through connection (Purvis et al., 2013).

Polyvagal theory, with its focus on the evolution of our autonomic stress response systems from immobilization (death feigning – freezing – at the neuroception of life threat) to mobilization (flight or fight) when we perceive danger, to social engagement when we neurocept safety (Dana, 2018; Porges, 2011) helps us understand some of the influence that SBBs can exert at the subconscious level. Importantly, the vagus nerve (attached at the base of the brain, very near the muscles of inner ear and the jaw) runs all the way down into the gut. Intentional use of our faces, tone of voice, and proxemics can co-regulate the escalated camper and defuse explosive situations.

In TraumaPlay, both exteroception (sensitivity to stimuli outside the body) and interoception (our felt experience of the inner workings of our bodies, including breath, heart rate, and digestion) are valuable tools in helping our clients know what they need to regulate (Salvato et al., 2020; Sherrington, 1906). The concept of "bigness and smallness in space" (Goodyear-Brown, 2019) and how each camper's perception of the space impacts their sense of felt safety is continually monitored. At Camp Nurture, all of the whole-group sessions happen in a shared room large enough to hold all campers and buddies. The Big Body Movement area, which invites big body engagement, was designed to meet both proprioceptive and vestibular (Kranowitz, 2005) needs through swinging, jumping, climbing, and crawling, while enhancing the trust relationship and relational risk taking between campers and their buddies. For example, crossing a slack line or being pulled along on a scooter board on their bellies, requires children with core trust issues to risk trusting their buddies in order to experience the competency surge of completing the slack line or zooming faster all the way across the room. Camp staff understand that while all campers could spend some time in the large group experiences and stretch their window of tolerance for social engagement, turn taking, and nurturing one another, there would also be many times that listening to their bodies would lead them to a smaller space to focus more on internal regulation or co-regulation with just a buddy. Thus, there are at least three separate cool down spaces pre-set at camp. Each of these spaces are set up in small rooms and include pillows, blankets, and some way to make even more contained spaces (a nylon tent or old sheets with which to create a small fort). Part of the magic of this kind of camp experience in which each camper has a buddy or two is that the buddy can move in and out of the larger group with the child.

The Structure of Camp Nurture

The daily schedule for Camp Nurture offers cyclical repetitions of experiences meant to enhance targeted neural growth. The components of the day are listed below.

Drop-Off-Attachment Script

Verbal and Physical Check-in: Each camper spends time connecting with their individually assigned SBB. This time allows the TraumaPlay trained adult to assess the camper's current state of regulation, connection, and executive function.

   Nurture Group: Adopted children can benefit from high doses of nurture. These groups offer a variety of activities grounded in the Theraplay model (Booth & Jernberg, 2010; Munns, 2017) and categorized along four dimensions of care (structure, engagement, nurture, challenge). Campers practice giving and receiving care. Activities such as feeding each other and offering band-aids to one another are offered to all campers. Campers also practice using their voice to negotiate getting needs met. They check in with the group using their Stress Engines, a tool developed as part of the Alert Program, an Occupational Therapy protocol used to help children learn about their own level of alertness (Williams & Shellenberger, 1996). The group leader asks, "Is your engine running too hot or too fast? Is your engine running to cold or too slow?" Campers learn to listen to what their bodies are telling them and to share their perceptions of their internal state with the group.

The Big Body Movement Circuit: This invites various forms of full-body, kinesthetic engagement. The space may resemble an occupational therapy floor and can contain obstacle course elements rearranged daily to offer different sorts of physical challenge. Campers take supported risks with their SBBs as experience competency surges, growing in confidence in themselves and with each other.

Snack Time: The pairing of relationship and resource, through feeding, is one of the earliest attachment enhancement behaviors.

LifeSkills Group: This group is normally anchored in a bibliotherapy resource that helps teach or normalize a feeling, contributing to the TraumaPlay goal of enhancing emotional literacy. This may include verbal practice of feelings expression, role play of feeling states with puppets, or exploration of what kinds of situations engender certain kinds of feelings. This group can also target a Life Skill that becomes important to the group as an outgrowth of the group process. Examples might include being gentle and kind, making a repair with a friend when a rupture has occurred, taking turns in game play, or mindfulness practice.

Outdoor Time: During this time the group can take a nature walk, engage in an outdoor scavenger hunt, go swimming, or participate in group challenges, such as creating a Stone Soup from berries, etc. it is important that SBBs stick close to their campers during this time to maintain felt safety and co-regulation in the outdoor environment. Occasionally, a camper may be too dysregulated to go outside.

Lunch: Campers have the opportunity to eat and talk together, practicing pro-social skills, often with just one other camper with the support of both camper's SBBs.

Nurture Group: A second group provides additional practice in using their voice, checking in with their bodies, and reflecting on the day's activities with their buddies and peers in a way that maximizes therapeutic learning.

Additional cycles of Big Body Movement Group and LifeSkills groups can be built in, depending on the needs of the campers. *The duration of each group can also be lengthened or shortened depending on attention span and developmental level of the camp participants.*

Case Example

Johnny was a four-year-old adopted child with a significant language delay, a sensory processing disorder, and an auto-immune disease that had kept him indoors most of his young life. Each morning Goodyear-Brown, as Camp Director, rehearsed an attachment script with Johnny's mom and dad, "Mom and dad, do I have permission to be the Safe Boss of Johnny today?" The parent would respond, "Yes, you have my permission." Goodyear-Brown would ask "May I also have your permission to give Johnny safe touches, like high fives and hugs when he needs them?" Johnny's parent would respond in the affirmative, offering specific insights about what kinds of touches felt most nurturing to him.

On the first day of camp, campers were given matching backpacks which they could decorate with their name and the name of their SBB. They then chose one of each tool laid about the room: a water bottle that required a strong sucking action to dispense water (the sucking reflex being a soothing mechanism), lollipops, bubble gum, fidgets, a Martian Popping Doll, and chewelry if they needed it. Campers had permission to request one of their individually approved snacks or drinks anytime their body told them they needed it. The concept being taught was how to check in with their bodies, know what their bodies were telling them, and then ask for what they needed. This was revolutionary for some of these children and for some of their parents as well. Since Johnny had only a handful of words at the start of camp, his SBBs focused on him using his words (simple phrases like "too noisy" or "I'm hungry" after checking in with his body).

Johnny and his SBB created a Stress Engine, (see Figure 6.1) and learned quickly that he needed frequent breaks away from the stimulation of the large group. After the first morning (when he refused to flush the toilet for fear of it hurting his ears) the staff provided him with noise cancelling headphones to wear whenever his body told him he needed them. During one of the last Nurture Group sessions, Goodyear-Brown asked the question, "If you have any superhero power what would it be?". It took 45 seconds for him to verbalize the answer, as he struggled through the bottom-up process of regulating himself internally, connecting with his SBB, and engaging his executive functioning skills to choose his answer and deliver it to the group. During that time, he remained in constant motion, rocking his body back and forth, touching his buddy's face, becoming distracted by the movement of others, and eventually refocusing before he declared in a booming voice, "My superpower is to be a tornado!". This big, marvelous voice and this even bigger, marvelous imaginative idea had been inside Johnny all along, it just took him more time to find it in the midst of the static. Johnny might not have done so in a regular classroom setting, as teachers frequently perceive delayed responses to questions as inattention, ignorance, or even defiance. Johnny's SBB learned quickly that he needed physical touch and patience in order to push through the sensory static in and around him. Waiting with support became a primary tool used with Johnny, and his confidence and ability to take verbal risks increased. Buddies used shared language, such as "gentle

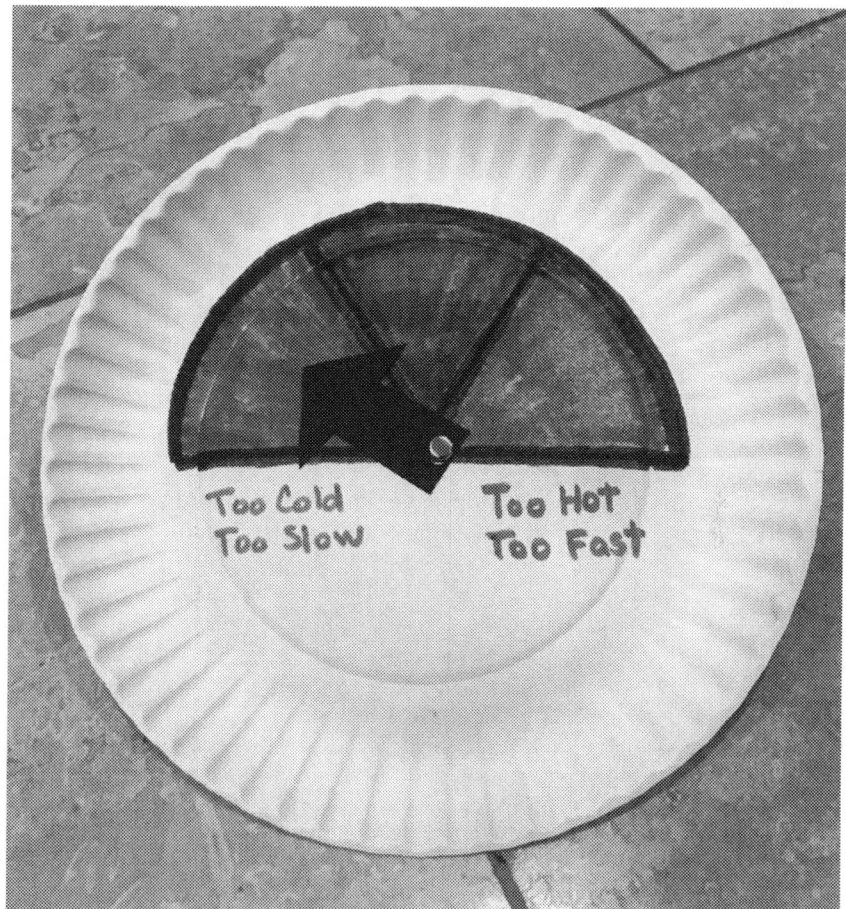

Figure 6.1 Example of a Stress Engine
Source: Photo courtesy of Paris Goodyear-Brown

and kind", "your body is letting me know that...", and "when you can ask me with your good asking words, I'm right here to give you a yes" were also valuable in building a culture of kindness between Johnny and the staff.

At the end of the first day of camp, Johnny became very dysregulated when it was time to leave. His disappointment was expressed through his body and he began to kick and hit. The escalation lasted 30 minutes. On the last day of camp, as his SBB walked with Goodyear-Brown, Johnny, and his parents to the car, he abruptly began to hit his dad. As his parents used the tools they had been taught to co-regulate him, he scrunched up his face, and said, "I will miss you". The violence stopped as soon as he was able to express his big feelings with connected caregivers. Johnny had experienced a large leap in his vocabulary during camp and left more regulated and more connected to his adoptive parents. Moreover, the parents reported feeling better equipped to be Safe Bosses for him moving forward.

Conclusion

Camp Nurture serves as another expression of the heart of TraumaPlay, using individual and group experiences to provide co-regulation through trauma-competent SBBs dozens of times throughout a day while ultimately expanding the window of tolerance for campers leveraging play as the vehicle for stretching cycles of up-regulation and down-regulation. Most importantly, parents' capacity to co-regulate their children more effectively is increased after experiencing Camp Nurture. Two key components of TraumaPlay, 1) soothing the physiology and 2) enhancing the role of parents as partners in co-regulation of their adoptive children, are supported by this immersive camp experience which highlights a unique way play therapy groups can be designed and implemented.

References

Adkins, T., Reisz, S., Doerge, K., & Nulu, S. (2020). Adverse Childhood Experience histories in foster parents: Connections to foster children's emotional and behavioral difficulties. *Child Abuse & Neglect*, 104, 104475.

Ainsworth, M. D. (1962). The effects of maternal deprivation: A review of findings and controversy in the context of research strategy. In M. D. Ainsworth, R. G. Andry, R. G. Harlow, & S. Lebovici. *Deprivation and maternal care: A reassessment of its effects.* Geneva: World Health Organization.

Almas, A. N., Papp, L. J., Woodbury, M. R., Nelson, C. A., Zeanah, C. H., & Fox, N. A. (2020). The impact of caregiving disruptions of previously institutionalized children on multiple outcomes in late childhood. *Child Development*, 91(1), 96–109.

Anthony, R. E., Paine, A. L., & Shelton, K. H. (2019). Adverse childhood experiences of children adopted from care: The importance of adoptive parental warmth for future child adjustment. *International Journal of Environmental Research and Public Health*, 16(12), 2212.

Banella, F. E. & Tronick, E. (2019). Mutual regulation and unique forms of implicit relational knowing. In G. Apter, E. Devouche, & M. Gratier (Eds.), *Early interaction and developmental psychopathology* (pp. 35–53). Springer, Cham.

Banella, F. E., Speranza, A. M., & Tronick, E. (2018). Mutual regulation and unique forms of implicit relational knowing. *Rassegna di Psicologia*, 35(3), 67–76.

Barnett, E. R., Jankowski, M. K., Butcher, R. L., Meister, C., Parton, R. R., & Drake, R. E. (2018). Foster and adoptive parent perspectives on needs and services: A mixed methods study. *The Journal of Behavioral Health Services & Research*, 45(1), 74–89.

Bellis, M. A., Hardcastle, K., Ford, K., Hughes, K., Ashton, K., Quigg, Z., & Butler, N. (2017). Does continuous trusted adult support in childhood impart life-course resilience against adverse childhood experiences – a retrospective study on adult health-harming behaviours and mental well-being. *BMC Psychiatry*, 17(1), 1–12.

Booth, P. B. & Jernberg, A. M. (2010). *Theraplay: Helping parents and children build better relationships through attachment-based play* (3rd ed.). Jossey Bass.

Carr, A. (2008). The effectiveness of family therapy and systemic interventions for child-focused problems. *Journal of Family Therapy*, 31, 3–45.

Cermak, S. A. & Daunhauer, L. A. (1997). Sensory processing in the post-institutionalized child. *American Journal of Occupational Therapy*, 51(7), 500–507.

Dana, D. A. (2018). *The Polyvagal theory in therapy: engaging the rhythm of regulation: Norton series on interpersonal neurobiology*. W. W. Norton & Company.

Doyle, C. & Cicchetti, D. (2017). From the cradle to the grave: The effect of adverse caregiving environments on attachment and relationships throughout the lifespan. *Clinical Psychology: Science and Practice*, 24(2), 203–217.

Gaskill, R. L. & Perry, B. D. (2012). Child sexual abuse, traumatic experiences, and their impact on the developing brain. In P. Goodyear-Brown (Ed.), *Handbook of child sexual abuse: Identification, assessment, and treatment* (pp. 29–47). Wiley.

Gaskill, R. L. & Perry, B. D. (2017). A neurosequential therapeutics approach to guided play, play therapy, and activities for children who won't talk. In C. A. Malchiodi & D. A. Crenshaw (Eds.), *What to do when children clam up in psychotherapy: Interventions to facilitate communication* (pp. 38–66). The Guilford Press.

Goodyear-Brown, P. (2010a). *Play therapy with traumatized children: A prescriptive approach*. Wiley.

Goodyear-Brown, P. (2010b). *The worry wars: An anxiety workbook for kids and their helpful adults*. Goodyear-Brown.

Goodyear-Brown, P. (2019). *Trauma and play therapy: Helping children heal*. Routledge.

Goodyear-Brown, P. (2021). *Parents as partners in child therapy: A clinician's guide*. The Guilford Press.

Gunnar M. (2001). Effects of early deprivation: Findings from orphanage-reared infants and children. In Nelson, C. A. & Luciana, M., (Eds.), *Handbook of developmental cognitive neuroscience* (pp. 617–629). MIT Press.

Hebb, D. (1949). *The organization of behavior*. Wiley.

Hoffman, K., Cooper, G., & Powell, B. (2017). *Raising a secure child: How circle of security parenting can help you nurture your child's attachment, emotional resilience, and freedom to explore*. Guilford Publications.

Hong, R. & Mason, C. M. (2016). Becoming a neurobiologically-informed play therapist. *International Journal of Play Therapy*, 25(1), 35–44.

Kay, J. (2009). Toward a neurobiology of child psychotherapy. *Journal of Loss and Trauma*, 14, 287–303.

Koss, K. J., Mliner, S. B., Donzella, B., & Gunnar, M. R. (2016). Early adversity, hypocortisolism, and behavior problems at school entry: A study of internationally adopted children. *Psychoneuroendocrinology*, 66, 31–38.

Kranowitz, C. S. (1998). *The out-of-sync child*. New York: Berkley Publishing Group.

Kranowitz, C. S. (2005). *The out-of-sync child: Recognizing and coping with sensory processing disorder*. The Berkley Publishing Group.

MacLean, D. P. (1990). *The triune brain in evolution: Role in paleocerebral functions*. Plenum Press.

McKirdy, G. C., Roughley, R. A., & McKirdy, S. A. (2019). From proving perfection to seeking support: The lived experiences of adoptive parents in Alberta. *Canadian Journal of Counselling and Psychotherapy*, 53(3), 276–295.

Munns, E. (2017). Group theraplay. In K. D. Buckwalter & D. Reed (Eds.), *Attachment theory in action: Building connections between children and parents* (pp. 105–120). Rowman and Littlefield.

Ogden, P., Minton. K., & Pain, C. (2006). *Trauma and the body: A sensorimotor approach to psychotherapy*. W. W. Norton and Company.

Perry, B. D. (2008). Child maltreatment: A neurodevelopmental perspective on the role of trauma and neglect in psychopathology. In T. P. Beauchaine & S. P. Hinshaw (Eds.), *Child and adolescent psychopathology* (pp. 93–128). Wiley.

Porges, S. W. (2011). *The polyvagal theory: Neurophysiological foundations of emotions, attachment, communication, and self-regulation (Norton Series on Interpersonal Neurobiology)*. W. W. Norton & Company.

Powell, B., Cooper, G., Hoffman, K., & Marvin, B. (2013). *The circle of security intervention: Enhancing attachment in early parent-child relationships*. Guilford publications.

Purvis, K., Cross, D., Dansereau, D., & Parris, S. (2013). Trust-based relational intervention (TBRI): A systemic approach to complex developmental trauma. *Child and Youth Services*, 34(4), 360–386.

Purvis, B. K., Cross, R. D., Federici, R., Johnson, D., & McKenzie, B. L. (2007). The Hope Connection: A therapeutic day camp for adopted and at-risk children with special socio-emotional needs. *Adoption and Fostering Quarterly Journal*, 31, 38–48.

Reilly, E. B. & Gunnar, M. R. (2019). Neglect, HPA axis reactivity, and development. *International Journal of Developmental Neuroscience*, 78, 100–108.

Salvato, G., Richter, F., Sedeño, L., Bottini, G., & Paulesu, E. (2020). Building the bodily self-awareness: Evidence for the convergence between interoceptive and exteroceptive information in a multilevel kernel density analysis study. *Human Brain Mapping*, 41(2), 401–418.

Schaefer, C. E. & Drewes, A. A. (2013). *The therapeutic powers of play: 20 core agents of change*. John Wiley & Sons.

Schore, A. N. (2000). Attachment and the regulation of the right brain. *Attachment & Human Development*, 2(1), 23–47.

Sherrington, C. S. (1906). *The integrative action of the nervous system*. Yale University Press.

Siegel, D. J. (2010). *Mindsight: The new science of personal transformation*. Bantam.

Siegel, D. J. & Bryson, T. P. (2012). *The whole-brain child: 12 revolutionary strategies to nurture your child's developing mind*. Bantam.

Siegel, D. J. & Hartzell, M. (2013). *Parenting from the inside out: How a deeper self- understanding can help you raise children who thrive*. Penguin.

Stewart, A. L., Field, T. A., & Echterling, L. G. (2016). Neuroscience and the magic of play therapy. *International Journal of Play Therapy*, 25(1), 4.

Tronick, E. Z. & Cohn, F. J. (1989). Emotions and emotional communication in infants. *American Psychologist*, 44(2), 112–119.

Wheeler, N. & Dillman Taylor, D. (2016). Integrating interpersonal neurobiology with play therapy. *International Journal of Play Therapy*, 25(1), 24–34.

Wilbarger, J., Gunnar, M., Schneider, M., & Pollak, S. (2010). Sensory processing in internationally adopted, post-institutionalized children. *Journal of Child Psychology and Psychiatry*, 51(10), 1105–1114.

Williams, M. S. & Shellenberger, S. (1996). The Alert Program™ for self-regulation. *American Occupational Therapy Association Sensory Integration Special Interest Section Newsletter*, 17, 1–3.

7 Our Village Play Therapy Groups

An Integrative Design for Both In-Person and Telehealth Settings

Monica Adimari Fyfe

Group play therapy is a powerful therapeutic format that structurally provides social connection amongst youth peers, instant and contingent social feedback in the here and now, vicarious learning from peers, and a normalization process that one is not alone with their psychological needs. In addition, "the group as a miniature society offers motivation and support for change, as well as a safe arena for testing new patterns of behavior" (Ginott, 1961, p. 13). Groups can also be fun and provide natural reinforcement for children within their sociocentric stage of development.

The mission at Our Village, a 501c3 non-profit agency in Redondo Beach, California, is to provide evidence-based play and social skills groups to children and teens. The clients served are both neurodivergent and neurotypical and have similar goals of decreasing social isolation or social rejection, improving social confidence, practicing perspective-taking and empathy for others, and improving self-awareness of one's own urges, thoughts, feelings, and behaviors.

This chapter shares the integrated design which has shown success at meeting the aforementioned types of client goals via a thoughtful combination of evidence-based approaches. This integrated design was created to: honor the whole child, follow progressive contextual behavioral sciences, utilize directive approaches, incorporate neurobiology, movement and sensory informed practices, be developmentally sensitive in supporting play, and bring in mentor peers to foster an inclusive and empathic community for all. The main approaches in this integrated design include: Acceptance and Commitment Therapy (ACT), Theraplay®, and Teaching Interactions (TI's). ACT provides a broad, behaviorally-based fluid structure that supports children and teens in their decision making, their self-awareness, their personalized goal-making and values development, and their understanding and acceptance of the way they think and feel related to others in their social world. Theraplay offers group members right-brain to right-brain attunement and attachment activities, simple social connecting games, co-regulation and synchronicity opportunities between other group members (and with the therapist), movement, challenge, and fun. Teaching Interactions offers the therapist and group members a systematic

DOI: 10.4324/9781003094531-7

and consistent way to effectively break down large, abstract social skills into age-appropriate, digestible steps, that can be rehearsed, internalized, and generalized in the natural group environment through peer-to-peer interactions towards mastery.

Group offerings at Our Village consist of both in-person and telehealth groups for older children and teens. Despite the practice of telehealth groups for children, there is a scarcity of research in this area. Therefore, throughout this chapter, the reader will find tips and accommodations that have successfully supported Our Village telehealth groups, as well as traditional in-person groups, for children and teens. The information shared is intended to help and inspire clinicians, play therapists, behavior analysts, and educators in meeting their own group's unique goals while applying similar group designs.

Research

Acceptance and Commitment Therapy with Children: A Play Therapy Approach

Traditional Applied Behavior Analysis (ABA) is considered the "1st wave" in behavioral therapies. It stems from a long line of empirically validated research on classical conditioning, operant conditioning, and social learning theory (Knell, 1995). A behavior therapist looks deeply into the function or purpose of a behavior and what it communicates by examining the context, settings, antecedents, and consequences that reinforce or maintain it. The goal is to possibly help shape a functionally equivalent replacement behavior over time. Regarding play, Knell (1995) noted that "play was used in behavioral play therapy, mainly as a way to engage the child in treatment, and thus was more of a means to an end rather than inherently valuable in and of itself" (p. 16).

With time, the behavior sciences have progressed to include Naturalistic Developmental Behavior Interventions (NDBI), described as a

> group of similar, empirically supported, autism interventions that represent the merging of applied behavioral and developmental sciences. NDBI's are implemented in natural settings, involve shared control between child and therapist, utilize natural contingencies, and use a variety of behavioral strategies to teach developmentally appropriate and prerequisite skills.
>
> (Schreibman et al., 2015, p. 2411)

NDBI approaches are well suited for toddlers through preschoolers. Our Village embeds NDBI principles and interventions in groups for the youngest group members.

The "2nd wave" of behavior therapies includes theories such as Cognitive Behavioral Therapy (CBT) and Rational Emotive Behavior Therapy

(REBT). "Cognitive Behavioral Therapy is the most researched, evidence-based and empirically-validated treatment approach that incorporates both cognitive and behavioral interventions in a systematic and goal-oriented manner" (Cavett & Drewes, 2019, p. 24). In CBT, Aaron Beck posited that irrational thoughts are the underlying reason for psychopathology, and subsequently impact feelings and behaviors (cognitive triangle). Irrational thoughts lead to negative affect or negative behavior. By changing one's thoughts, feelings and behaviors can change as well. In CBT, the client is involved in creating their goals and treatment plan (Cavett & Drewes, 2019).

Cavett and Drewes (2019) noted that children under eight years old do not have abstract thinking or language abilities necessary for CBT. Consequently, Cognitive Behavior Play Therapy (CBPT) was developed to "provide a theoretical framework based on cognitive-behavioral principles and integrates these in a developmentally sensitive way" (Knell, 1995, p. 43). Cavett and Drewes (2019) share that "CBPT has not been extensively researched, although it has been extensively utilized and written about" (p. 24).

Harris (2019) shared that the "3rd wave" of the most modern behavioral therapies brought Acceptance and Commitment Therapy (ACT), along with Dialectical Behavior Therapy (DBT), Mindfulness-based Cognitive Therapy (MBCT), Functional Analytic Psychotherapy (FAP), and others, from a school of behaviorism called functional contextualism. These therapies all have a major emphasis on acceptance, mindfulness, and compassion.

ACT is rooted in Relational Frame Theory (RFT), which is a behavior analytic account of language and cognitions. There are relational frames of language that people derive for themselves with helpful and unhelpful connections. "ACT and RFT focuses on how and why language occurs, rather than the way it looks or sounds" (Dixon & Paliliunas, 2018, p. 21).

Both CBT and ACT utilize behavior contingency management. A main difference between CBT and ACT is the conceptualization of how to interact with one's negative thoughts or cognitions. A goal of CBT is to change or stop one's negative thoughts from occurring in order to produce affective change. In comparison, a goal of ACT is to accept all thoughts positive and negative, notice they are there without a goal to change them, while staying in contact with the present moment. Acceptance of all thoughts, feelings, and memories in both positive and negative forms are described in ACT as a normal part of life. An ACT clinician helps clients develop psychological and behavioral flexibility to pursue desired experiences with committed action steps towards one's values.

Mindfulness practice is a big part of ACT that allows awareness of the present moment (not past or future), with nonjudgmental observation. Metaphors are also important in ACT in noticing and untangling the meaning for stories one keeps. The paths to arriving at improved psychological flexibility are described through six core processes often depicted in a visual diagram called a Hexaflex. The processes include: Present Moment

Awareness, Acceptance, Defusion, Self-As-Context, Values, and Committed Action. Research regarding ACT has focused on Hexaflex processes, as well as the effectiveness of ACT, on various populations. For example, Enoch and Dixon (2017) researched children with ADHD that strived to enhance their ability to contact the present moment. This involved shifting attention to the here and now with both internal and external stimuli present. Results demonstrated that participation in the use of an ACT curriculum for children helped increase their attention outcomes.

There have been two meta-analyses done on the effectiveness of ACT for children. Swain et al. (2015) concluded that studies showed emerging promise but not enough studies with scientific rigor were available to conclude ACT was effective in children. Fang and Ding (2020) looked at 14 International Randomized Control Trials prior to 2018. A Randomized Control Trial (RCT) is a scientific experiment or intervention study that aims to reduce sources of bias by randomly assigning participants into an experimental group or a control group. As the study is conducted, the only expected difference between the control and experimental groups is the outcome variable being studied. The findings of Fang and Ding (2020) indicated that:

> ACT is more effective than Treatment as Usual and untreated groups in treating anxiety, depression and other mental and behavioral disorders, while not superior to traditional CBT. There was no difference between ACT and traditional CBT in their effectiveness of both improving negative psychological factors and behaviors in children.
>
> (p. 229)

Although there are some promising results, there is a need for continued research in evaluating the effectiveness and processes of change within ACT interventions for children.

Dixon and Paliliunas (2018) created AIM (Accept, Identify, Move) for children as a full year social and emotional school curriculum that incorporates the ACT Hexaflex processes, mindfulness, and behavior analysis together. Here is an example of a scenario where Dixon and Palilunas (2018) demonstrate ACT:

> Imagine a child is afraid to ride a bike, an activity they really care about- being active and independent. He will not try it saying I'm scared. Applying ACT, one might respond No you're not scared... you're James! You're just having the thought that you're scared. What does it mean to you to ride that bike? Are you committed to trying, even if it's a little bit scary?
>
> (p. 42)

Dixon and Paliliunas (2018) also shared some tips on how to adapt ACT for children since many concepts can be abstract and require advanced language. These tips included: make the lesson metaphors more concrete by physicalizing them, utilize experiential activities, and translate the concepts into child friendly language.

Theraplay

Theraplay has been recognized by the Association for Play Therapy as a historically significant play therapy approach for children and is evidence-based. Theraplay was created by Ann Jernberg in 1967 in a Chicago Head Start program (Booth & Jernberg, 2010). She was mandated to find a way to serve the mental health needs of hundreds of children who needed help. She created a program with activities modelled on the healthy, playful patterns of interactions between parent and child and borrowed elements from the work of Austin DesLauriers and Viola Brody in developing Theraplay (Booth & Jernberg, 2010, p. xxiii).

Booth and Jernberg (2010) shared that "although DesLauriers recognized the positive findings of behavioral therapists, such as Lovaas, for improving the skills of a child with autism, he believed that treatment must focus on increasing the child's social and emotional connection with others" (p. 303). Thereafter, with the influence of DesLauriers' relationship-based approach at its core, Theraplay is being used internationally to help children build connections, including children with autism (Booth & Jernberg, 2010).

Booth and Lindaman (2019) noted that Theraplay targets the lower and mid-brain areas for children with repetitive and rhythmic activities. Theraplay fills in gaps of developmental arrests by working from the bottom up and by providing new experiences of mastery evidence for the developing brain. In addition, sessions utilizing this therapeutic model are designed to provide an intermix between up-regulating play and movement activities with down-regulating focus. Soothing and nurturing play activities gently expand a child's window of tolerance, including their ceiling and floor, towards more optimal arousal levels over time. Booth and Lindaman (2019) also shared that these processes apply to group Theraplay as well, where the focus shifts from traditional caregiver to child interactions to therapist to group member, and member to member connections.

Teaching Interactions

The Autism Partnership method of teaching social skills groups is a systematic, individualized, and behaviorally-based approach. Teaching Interactions is a commonly used intervention used to teach social skills (Leaf et al., 2020). First developed by Minikin and colleagues (1976), Autism Partnership adapted the use of Teaching Interactions successfully in breaking down and teaching social skills to their group members. The Teaching Interaction (TI) procedure is a multi-component intervention consisting of six steps (Leaf et al., 2020):

1   Labeling the target behavior (*in age-appropriate terms*).
2   Providing a meaningful rationale of why the learner should engage in the target behavior (*gathered by members and therapist*).
3   Describing the steps of the target skill.
4   Modeling of the target skill (*by the therapists, right and wrong ways are shown*).
5   Role-Play of the skill (*by the group members, only the right way is shown*).
6   Offering feedback throughout (*during intervention and catching a child showing the skill during unstructured and more natural parts of group to promote generalization*).

Research from Leaf et al. (2012) showed that when comparing teaching interactions to social stories in mastering novel social skills,

> ...the teaching interaction procedure resulted in mastery of all 18 skills taught, across the 6 participants. Social stories, in the same amount of teaching sessions, resulted in mastery of 4 of the 18 social skills taught, across the 6 participants.

(p. 281)

In addition, participants showed an added benefit of displaying increased generalization of the social skills learned from teaching interactions, with both familiar adults and peers.

Integration of Acceptance and Commitment Therapy: A Group Approach

Applying principles of Acceptance and Commitment Therapy for Play Therapy provides a developmentally sensitive framework to providing ACT interventions to children and teens. An important part of ACT is helping a client reflect and discriminate what values in life are the most meaningful to them. It is an individualized response that changes over time in different life stages. By engaging children in ACT principles early on through the language of play, it is hoped that children can grow to broaden their capacity towards psychological flexibility across their lifetime.

Once values are established, another important process in ACT is making mindful choices. Therapists can utilize the Choice Point metaphor (Harris, 2019) to support group members in this process. Choice Point in ACT is a visual way to map out a problem with a two-arrow diagram. The therapist uses this visual to help their client reflect on the choices they are considering, either by showing movement towards their values or movement away from the values one cares about.

In telehealth play therapy, a group intervention to facilitate Choice Point is called *Towards and Away*. After explaining Choice Point to the group members, the therapist selects a hypothetical problem scenario with context pertinent to the age and goals of the group, (e.g., scenarios based on fear and anxiety, friendship skills, teasing). The therapist can share these scenarios in playful, digital ways including online wheel spinners of problems, online coin flippers, showing memes or popular movie clips of the problem, or sharing a fictional advice columnist blog such as "Dear Aunt Blabby" who needs the help of the *expert* group members.

After the problem is shared, the therapist states the values of the hypothetical child, the problem, and the choice that was made. Group members can then vote between two choices with their whole bodies in a non-verbal way: A) if group members feel the child in the hypothetical scenario made a choice that brought them closer "towards their values" they would move their faces and eyes exaggeratingly close to their web cameras, or B) if the child made a choice that took them "further away" from contacting their values, group members would scoot their faces and bodies far, far away from their cameras to show their vote.

Group members have fun getting a chance to play with body proximity and movement surrounding their cameras. Also, it clearly stands out when a member does not agree with the majority vote and that gives the group a great chance to process together and possibly uncover potentially self-defeating thoughts and behaviors of some members.

A helpful book and ACT program, written for therapists to adapt ACT for teens, is called, "The Thriving Adolescent," by Joseph Ciarrochi and Louise Hayes (2015). Here the authors use a Discoverer-Noticer-Advisor-Values (DNA-V) model and a related DNA-V compass to help synthesize and present a developmentally appropriate system to help older children and teens digest the larger and more abstract concepts of ACT.

The DNA-V compass template has been a helpful tool in both traditional in-person and telehealth play therapy groups at Our Village. They are fun and easy to make and require minimal art materials including paper, an optional thumb tack for added movement in the center dial, and some markers. This expressive arts intervention has been a common overarching group theme each week. Children are encouraged to stay in the present moment and attend to the signals they receive from three key areas of the compass: 1) The Discover: to expand our ways of taking chances in the world, how we explore and take risks, 2) The Noticer: to detect internal, physical, psychological, social, and environmental events inside us and in our social world and 3) The Advisor: to notice what rules or language come up that can be *helpful or not so helpful*. Lastly, all three areas and subsequent life choices are balanced by the center of the compass, represented by personalized life values, which in ACT leads one closer to goals of psychological flexibility and vitality.

Thereafter, for both in-person and telehealth group play therapy, a therapist can model a mantra or group chant such as "Follow your north" or "Follow your arrow". After hearing a Choice Point scenario, members take physical steps and *"bravely march towards their north"*, in either home or clinic settings. In doing so their steps are a symbol for taking small, committed actions towards their values, even when things are hard. Images of the compass, videos and parent handouts can be found on the authors website at: www.thrivingadolescent.com.

Integration of Theraplay: A Group Approach

In traditional in-person groups at Our Village, Theraplay activities are woven into the schedule to offer group members and leaders needed movement, touch, and peer-connecting breaks. Theraplay's joyful, synchronistic, and up/down regulating play can be a respite for group members from the more abstract ACT concepts or behavior and cognitive skill building practice of Teaching Interactions.

"Virtual Theraplay groups can be challenging for therapists because of the usual focus on in-person presence, tuning into subtleties, therapeutic touch, and physicality" (F. Peacock, personal communication, January 7, 2021). Peacock shared some helpful reflections and modifications for telehealth Theraplay groups. Games that work best involve large visual and physical changes and movements. Subtle games with tracking eye movement or changes in tone or rhythm such as group singing are challenging because of "lag time" across tech and Wi-Fi delays which may impact the therapist's goal of group synchronicity.

However, some wonderful Theraplay activities can be embedded into telehealth groups that involve obvious, independent large movement and vocal changes (over joint, coordinated movements). F. Peacock (personal communication, January 7, 2021) described a game to play when one group member is not tuned in and has low arousal. Here the therapist does not want to disrupt the momentum of the entire group that is doing well. Our Village has adapted this game and lovingly dubbed it, *Secret Agent Pictionary*.

In *Secret Agent Pictionary*, the therapist playfully suggests a game to the group where they intermittently initiate private chats to group members. When the therapist notices one child needing some arousal and structure, the therapist purposefully targets that child with a special private message in the chat to draw a simple picture (such as a star) and present it to the group by holding up their paper for all to see. The rest of the group members need only to quickly shout out the name of the drawing, as they were already engaged and tuned in. The group has fun, moves on, and thereafter the child who drew the picture is now more engaged without adult feedback or disrupting the flow of the group.

Below are some additional Theraplay activities that have been reported by A. Bushala, (personal communication, December 31, 2020) which translate well via group telehealth.

- *Imaginary Ball Toss – call a child's name and tell them what type of "ball" you will be pretending to throw to them. They catch it as the thing you tossed and then change it before calling the next person's name and tossing back (i.e., football, fire ball, medicine ball, snowball, water balloon, raw egg).*

- *Any call and response song (Tootie Tah, Cuddly Koalas, Go Bananas, Penguin Song).*
- *Simon Says, Add to It, Peanut Butter and Jelly, Copy My Move, Freeze Dance.*

Therapists can also find these descriptions and over 50 Theraplay Activities for Telehealth at: https://theraplay.org/product/theraplay-activities-for-telehealth/.

Integration of Teaching Interactions: A Group Approach

A play therapist can add a developmentally appropriate spin on teaching interactions with play props such as movie clippers, a peer yelling "Lights, camera, action". and another peer using symbolic play to record the dyad with an imaginary video camera. All of these techniques have translated well to both in-person and telehealth play groups. The main challenge for telehealth groups is that teaching interactions cannot involve large role-play movements off-camera. Therapists should adjust their play and social goals for this and plan accordingly with smaller movements and similar adaptations. Play therapists can also add Google slides of a movie company and utilize puppets, action figures, or comic strip drawings for behavioral and cognitive rehearsals as well. Group members should be encouraged to reflect on perspective-taking of their peers and empathy targets throughout these interventions.

Formation of Our Village Telehealth Play Therapy Groups

Getting Started

A therapist should ask themselves important questions before making the bridge to a tele-play process. Mellenthin (2020) proposed the following therapist self-reflection questions: "Is this client developmentally appropriate for play therapy-based, telehealth services? Has the therapist acquired the education to understand the clinical guidelines available for providing telehealth services using models of play therapy?" (p. 20). These reflective questions serve as important considerations for a therapist before implementing telehealth services.

Practical Considerations

Therapists will want to select the appropriate virtual platform to meet their setting needs. An essential criterion for the video-conferencing platform is to offer HIPAA compliance through a signed, mutual Business Associate Agreement (BAA) between the video-conferencing platform and the therapist. A telehealth informed consent form and release and liability agreement form should be reviewed and signed by clients, prior to starting treatment. This includes information provided in a language that clients understand, an emergency plan for safety, and back-up plan for technology concerns. Therapists should review this information and answer any questions before clients consent to virtual group therapy services for their child, and their related parent education telehealth sessions. Therapists should consult with their state licensing board to ensure all requirements are met.

Selection of Group Members and Group Make-Up

At Our Village, we determined that telehealth groups were most effective for older children, ages 8–12 years old, based on their focus, cognition, and language abilities. At this age, a duration of 45–90 minutes is developmentally appropriate. A special asset to telehealth groups is that it can be offered to potential members nationally, if they reside where the therapist is licensed professionally. This opens up a robust group member pool to find a "goodness of fit" between members and provides broader access to remote families in need.

At Our Village, mentor peers are also included as volunteers with both in-person and telehealth groups. Mentors receive training about neurodiversity and what to expect in group. Thereafter, the mentors are treated as regular members of the group. They are not mini-teachers or mini-parents to other members. They are involved in the same fun games, skill development, and homework and they receive feedback when needed. Most of all, mentors are also learning how best to interact with peers that are neurodivergent, gain leadership skills, empathy, and increased self-confidence.

Behavior Plan and Limit Setting

Parents and group members should be primed ahead of time about the therapist's plan of limit setting to protect group integrity and ensure feelings of safety and respect. It is important for the therapist to anticipate and set limits only as needed, after allowing members a chance to resolve issues between themselves, for both in-person and telehealth groups.

The use of grounding touch for redirection or inviting a child to walk away for a break to a chill zone (sensory calming area) are additional strategies therapists can utilize for in-person groups. However, these recommendations cannot occur over a screen via telehealth, so therapists should plan for modifications.

M. Winstead (personal communication, January 11, 2021) shared her modifications when conducting telehealth Theraplay groups,

In a telehealth group format, the therapist has more limitations because placing a traditional hand on a child's shoulder, or body proximity of walking towards a child, cannot occur. Instead via telehealth, the therapist can make a plan to provide each child with an index card of skills to organize oneself, such as taking care of one's needs for hunger, thirst, rest, taking a breath, asking for help or a break. If a child becomes disorganized during the group, the therapist can ask the child to turn their camera off briefly, try some organizing skills from their card, report in the chat what they tried to the therapist, and re-join the group when more regulated. Caregivers are also available at home to help. These organizing skills are modelled and practiced ahead of time in group, so children feel more prepared to attempt self-regulation skills, on or off camera.

Group Rules

Instead of adults creating the rules for the group, a therapist can use the Socratic Method to ask its members to reflect on "what group rules are important to you to feel safe and have fun in group?" Then, create a common agreement of what the guiding rules should be, produced by everyone's collective values. A fun visual such as a team poster for in-person groups, or a Google slide for telehealth groups, affirms these rules to the members. Examples of collaborative rules may include: be respectful and use friendly words, do not hurt others, activities can change, and we are flexible, no tech out (during in-person groups), no spamming or private messaging in the chat (for telehealth).

Case Example of a Telehealth Play Therapy Group at Our Village

In a telehealth group that was held once per week for 8 weeks, six group members ages 8–11 were brought together based on their common language and cognition abilities, ability to focus online with limited caregiver support, and similar overlapping goals. These goals included taking the perspectives of others, good sportsmanship, feelings and values exploration, and improving their social confidence to take brave risks in front of their peers.

This group was run by a lead therapist and a co-facilitator (therapy intern), with two children volunteering as mentors weekly, comprising of eight group members. The lead therapist assessed for common interests and affinities within the group and embedded them throughout the sessions to keep a natural engagement of the members. Parents were supported by weekly email summaries, and virtual group parent education meetings.

Therapists mailed the group members important templates of the DNA-V Compass, character trading card template, and parent handouts. Also, fun small toys were mailed, such as a mini "Etch a Sketch" for *Secret Agent Pictionary*, spinning tops for a good sportsmanship Teaching Interaction and more. Mailing a few items helps reduce stress on families with low resources, helps keep group members prepared for telehealth interventions, and engages clients to anticipate the fun ahead when receiving a special package in the mail.

During the initial stages, members created group rules collaboratively and voted on a team name. Group homework included creating *Character Trading Cards* to reflect on their imagined powers and values and a *Mystery Box* of a personal item to share later in group. During session, members also worked on a Defusion exercise of playing with the power of feeling words, to use with the *Smash-Up*'s activity. With a tri-folded paper, members came up with funny new combos by folding words together such as: "smad" (sad and mad), "wonxious" (worried and anxious), and "sited" (scared and excited). New feeling words were flexible and inclusive instead of overwhelming and absolute.

During this session, the children learned valuable social skills via Teaching Interactions of how to set up a virtual playdate and ways to be a good sport. Virtual playdates were assigned soon after the whole group practice, where members could generalize game play outside of session in pairs. Theraplay games of *Imaginary Ball Toss, What's Different*, and *Simon Says* were utilized throughout the time together for movement and group connection.

As treatment evolved, each group member demonstrated improvement towards their goals. Group members had learned self-regulation coping strategies through experiential activities in group of what felt good to them. This included breathing, muscle tightening, singing, or taking a break. Members drew symbols of these adopted strategies on their personalized "coping cards" which became a transitional item for generalization once group was completed. On the last day of group, a Graduation Day was held that included music, zoom filter fun, a BYOC (Bring your own cupcake) to celebrate, a Talent Show theme, and a prize selection (mailed after group).

Conclusion

The Our Village integrative model of play therapy groups has shown to be effective, developmentally sensitive, neurobiology informed, and encompassing of a child's mind, body, feelings, behaviors, spirit, self, and social self. This model is rooted in science; it is progressive and flexible in its core adjusting to modern research findings. This integration has also proved to be effective with both telehealth and traditional in-person play therapy groups for older children. It strives to be neurodivergent affirming and inclusive for all. Future research is needed to delineate which variables are significant for therapists to consider in telehealth group play therapy to show a positive effect in group member's progress. Additionally, research pinpointing the processes of ACT that are most applicable and effective for children across various diagnoses as a proposed trans-diagnostic approach would be beneficial.

References

Booth, P. B. & Jernberg, A. M. (2010). *Theraplay: Helping parents and children build better relationships through attachment-based play.* Jossey-Bass.

Booth, P. & Lindaman, S. (2019, September) Attachment Theory and Theraplay. *Play Therapy Magazine,* 14(3), 14–16.

Cavett, A. & Drewes, A. (2019, September). Cognitive Behavioral Play Therapy. *Play Therapy Magazine,* 14(3), 24–26.

Ciarrochi, J. & Hayes, L. (2015). *The Thriving adolescent: Using acceptance and commitment therapy and positive psychology to help teens manage emotions, achieve goals and build connection.* New Harbinger.

Dixon, M. R. & Paliliunas, D. (2018). *AIM Accept, Identify, Move: A behavior analytic curriculum for social-emotional development in children.* Shawnee Scientific Press, LLC.

Enoch, M. R. & Dixon, M. R. (2017). The use of a child-based acceptance and commitment therapy curriculum to increase attention. *Child & Family Behavior Therapy,* 39(3), 200–224. doi:10.1080/07317107.2017.1338454.

Fang, S. & Ding, D. (2020). A meta-analysis of the efficacy of acceptance and commitment therapy for children. *Journal of Contextual Behavioral Science,* 15, 225–234.

Ginott, H. (1961). *Group psychotherapy with children: The theory and practice of play therapy.* McGraw-Hill.

Harris, R. (2019). *ACT made simple: An easy-to-read primer on acceptance and commitment therapy.* New Harbinger.

Knell, S. M. (1995). *Cognitive-Behavioral play therapy.* Jason Aronson Inc.

Leaf, J., Oppenheim-Leaf, M., Call, N., Sheldon, J., Sherman, J., Taubman, M., Mceachin, J., Dayharsh, J., & Leaf, R. (2012). Comparing the teaching interaction procedure to social stories for people with autism. *Journal of Applied Behavior Analysis,* 45(2), 281–298.

Leaf, J., Milne, C., Leaf, J., Rafuse, J., Cihon, J., Ferguson, J., Oppenheim-Leaf, M., Leaf, R., Mceachin., J., & Mountjoy, T. (2020). *The autism partnership method: Social skills groups.* Different Roads to Learning, Inc.

Mellenthin, C. (2020, December). The therapeutic powers of play at work in the age of telehealth. *Play Therapy Magazine,* 15(4), 20–22.

Minikin, N., Braukmann, C. J., Minkin, B. L., Timbers, G. D., Timbers, B. J., & Fixsen, D. L. (1976). The social validation and training of conversational skills. *Journal of Applied Behavior Analysis,* 9, 127–139.

Schreibman, L., Dawson, G., Stahmer, A. C., Landa, R., Rogers, S. J., McGee, G. G., Kasari, C., Ingersoll, B., Kaiser, A. P., Bruinsma, Y., McNerney, E., Wetherby, A., & Halladay, A. (2015). Naturalistic developmental behavioral interventions: Empirically validated treatments for autism spectrum disorder. *Journal of Autism and Developmental Disorders,* 45(8), 2411–2428.

Swain, J., Hancock, K., Dixon, A., & Bowman, J. (2015). Acceptance and commitment therapy for children: A systematic review of intervention studies. *Journal of Contextual Behavioral Science,* 4(2), 73–85.

Part II
Clinical Settings

8   Group Play Therapy in Schools

Timothy "T.J." Schoonover and Kristi Perryman

Play therapy has been established as the most developmentally appropriate way to work with elementary age children and has a history of use in clinical and school settings (Landreth et al., 2009; Landreth, 2012; Perryman, 2016). Due to the high number of students to mental health professional (MHP) ratio, group play therapy is an efficient way to address mental health needs in schools for multiple students at once, while simultaneously creating an environment to learn and practice new skills that they can apply in the outside world (Yalom & Leszcz, 2005). This chapter will cover the rationale and considerations for group play therapy in schools. Furthermore, this chapter will discuss Child-Centered Group Play Therapy (CCGPT) and provide readers with a case study of CCGPT in schools.

Why Group Play Therapy in Schools?

There is an increasing need for evidence-based developmentally appropriate interventions to treat the growing number of students in schools with mental health concerns. The U.S. Department of Health & Human Services Administration for Children and Families Office of Planning, Research and Evaluation (2010) reported that as early as Head Start (early intervention for low-income families), children had more behavioral issues in the classroom leading to negative impacts on the stress levels of teachers, staff, and overall learning. O'Connell et al. (2009) highlighted children's mental health disorders as a public health issue in the US and found that anywhere from 13–20% of children have had a mental health disorder. The impact of systemic racism and microaggressions experienced by minoritized students on a daily basis has created additional mental health concerns (Post et al., 2019). The long-term effects of these issues not being treated has dire implications as children grow into adulthood such as dropping out of high school, increased risk for incarceration, difficulty keeping a job, and health issues (Copeland et al., 2015). Early intervention, such as play therapy services provided by trained MHPs in school

DOI: 10.4324/9781003094531-8

settings are a viable option for preventing these early mental health concerns from following students into adulthood.

The Center for Disease Control and Prevention (2013) reported that the earlier mental health issues can be identified and addressed, it could result in improved academic success for students. Having mental health issues can inhibit a student's social, emotional, and academic development. These early mental health issues that arise can be addressed by MHPs through the use of counseling services, with play therapy being the most developmentally appropriate. Simon et al. (2015) reported that 53% of 6–11-year-old children with mental health issues received treatment and 18.6% of them received the treatment in school from MHPs. Providing these services at school is important due to the need and ability to treat students in their natural environment and that the school represents a microcosm of society (Perryman, 2016). It has been suggested that schools take action steps to provide services to students and families with school-based services and meet the important goal of eliminating racial/ethnic and socioeconomic disparities in the ability to access mental healthcare services (Department of Health and Human Services, 2000).

It has been posited that utilization of play therapy by MHPs in schools is appropriate due to the accessibility and familiarity with students (Perryman, 2016). One of the main MHPs in schools is the school counselor. The school counselor is often the central person responsible for providing direct counseling services to students as well as referring them to other MHPs associated with the school. They are typically familiar with all of the students and have relationships with teachers and parents. The professional school counselor's access to and familiarity with students and their families ensure groups can be a resourceful avenue for play therapy trained MHPs to address multiple students' mental health issues.

There is a myriad of reasons that schools are ideal for group play therapy. The use of play therapy is the most developmentally appropriate approach for working with elementary age students. CCPGT has shown to be beneficial for increasing both receptive and expressive language skills, decreasing anxiety and suicide risk, improving externalizing, internalizing and total behavior problems, as well as improving self-concept, negative mood, competence, and negative self-esteem related to depression and anxiety (Ray & McCullough, 2016). Additionally, Ray (2011) suggested seven benefits to group play therapy: 1) provides a comfort level for the child, 2) better child participation, 3) vicarious and induced catharsis, 4) vicarious and direct learning, 5) therapist opportunity for observation, 6) reality testing and limit setting, and 7) positive interactions. Although none of these specifically mention academic development, they overlap with social-emotional development, which impacts academic development, and is typically the primary focus of schools. Although schools can be an ideal setting to utilize group play therapy, there are considerations before implementation.

Considerations for Group Play Therapy in Schools

Whether it is a school counselor, school social worker, or school-based counselor, the MHPs first consideration is advocacy. MHPs who provide group play therapy will need to educate and advocate school administrators regarding the purpose and goals of play therapy, specifically group play therapy. Landreth (2012) suggests that elementary schools are an ideal location to provide play therapy, because of their focus on academic and social-emotional development. Additionally, he emphasized that it is not a question of *if* play therapy should be used in elementary schools, but *how* it is used. There have been multiple articles and books written about special considerations when developing programs incorporating the use of play therapy in schools (Perryman, 2010; 2016; Ray, 2010; 2011; Trice-Black et al., 2013).

Perryman (2010; 2016) suggests that a roadblock of implementing play therapy in schools could be school administrators. It is suggested for the MHP to educate teachers and administrators about the goals and purpose of play therapy through presentations and conversations (Perryman, 2016). The conversations about the role play therapy in schools are important and should begin during the initial job interview. Ray (2010; 2011) recommends when discussing the goals and purpose of play therapy in schools to connect it back to academic development of students. Additionally, providing school administrators with current research and informational material on the efficacy of play therapy in schools can help with this process.

Another consideration when using play therapy in schools is advocating for space (Perryman, 2010; 2016; Ray, 2010; 2011; Trice-Black et al., 2013). The MHP might need to advocate for a dedicated space for play therapy and appropriate toys. Typically, space is limited in schools and finding an appropriate and confidential room for play therapy can be difficult. Play therapy is recommended to be completed in a room with white walls, shelves for toys, non-carpeted floor, a sink, a bathroom, table and chairs, plenty of space for movement, and lots of toys (Landreth, 2012). However, finding a space that meets all these specifications in a school is difficult. Most MHPs have to move around a building to complete their play therapy sessions with students. For this reason, it is recommended they create a portable play therapy tote, which will be discussed later in this chapter. Advocating with administrators for a dedicated space and investment in appropriate play therapy toys will be crucial for the success of group play therapy.

An additional consideration when using play therapy in schools is the inclusion of teachers in the process. Teachers spend upwards of eight hours a day with students and can be the first to recognize potential mental health issues. It is important that teachers understand the purpose and goals of play therapy. It is recommended that conversations and in-service trainings be led by the MHPs with school staff to educate them on the efficacy of play therapy (Perryman, 2010; 2016; Ray, 2010; 2011). Additionally, teachers can provide invaluable feedback on how students are progressing before, during, and after treatment. If possible, it is recommended that MHPs have teachers complete standardized assessments to assess if play therapy is assisting them in the classroom. This can be done by utilizing a pre-post assessment before and after the play therapy intervention. This can provide valuable information to the MHP. Perryman (2016) suggested that it is important to collect data to show the impact of the group and share this information with administrators and stakeholders to advocate for the efficacy of play therapy in schools.

Another consideration of using play therapy in schools is connecting with and getting consent from guardians. It is unethical for a school counselor to begin individual or group play therapy with students without obtaining consent from their guardians. A school-based counselor might have additional steps to complete before working with a student based on their agency's policies.

In addition to the previous considerations, the last recommendation would be for MHPs to identify areas to be addressed in groups through a needs assessment. A brief needs assessment can be created with common issues of elementary students such as social emotional development, academics, bullying, etc. There should also be a fill-in-the blank for areas not addressed. The needs assessment should provide a space for teachers to indicate ideal times for students to participate in groups. It should also have a place for teachers to refer specific students who could benefit from group play therapy. The needs assessment should be given at multiple points throughout the school year. Around four weeks into the first semester is an ideal time for the first needs assessment because students have become settled and mental health and academic issues would be more apparent. Additionally, the needs assessment should be given at the end of the first and second semesters.

Creating a screening process is also an important element for groups. Sweeney (2011) provided some recommendations for play therapy groups. First, he recommends that completing individual play therapy, even one session, can be helpful for screening for appropriateness for a group. Second, that the group have a balance of genders and avoiding one gender having a majority. Third, that the MHP use their judgement on having participants who have experienced the same event or a part of the same population. Lastly, he recommends that participants be no more than 12 months apart in age. For school-based play therapy groups it would be within one grade of each other; however, most school-based play therapy involves students from the same grade.

Another point of consideration is the number of participants in a group. It is recommended that there be one facilitator per three participants. If there are two facilitators, there should be no more than six participants. If there are too many participants, it makes it difficult for the facilitator to be attuned to the entire group and limits the space in which participants can move around. Sweeney (2011) recommended that the younger the population, the smaller the group size.

Returning students to class after the group will need some attention. Children should return to the classroom in a non-dysregulated state, so they are not disruptive in class. Participants could become dysregulated towards the end of the group session or might have extra energy from the group. This can be addressed by completing deep breathing or other grounding exercises before they return to class and participate without disruption.

A final consideration is confidentiality. When a student is getting pulled from class by the MHPs, almost all their classmates will know where they are going. It is important to coordinate with the teacher on the best times for the group and how to discretely pull a student from class. A specific confidentiality consideration for school groups is that group members might not keep what is talked about in the group confidential. This can be addressed during the first group when discussing confidentiality with the students, stressing to all the participants that group content is not to be shared outside of the group meetings.

The MHPs must be trained in group counseling along with the play therapy modality they choose to utilize. Child-Centered Play Therapy (CCPT) is one of the most researched and commonly taught play therapy modalities (Lambert et al., 2007; Yee et al., 2019). Thus, we posit that CCGPT could be easy to implement by MHPs in schools.

Research/Theory

Child-Centered Group Play Therapy (CCGPT) is developed from Child-Centered Play Therapy (CCPT) and its person-centered philosophy of change. CCPT is known for its non-directiveness, focus on the relationship, and the use of specific skills to assist children in their social emotional development and address their mental health issues. CCGPT has been implemented for over 50 years and used in many settings. It has been posited that focusing on creating a safe environment in a client-centered group creates the conditions for clients to choose to self-actualize or not (Berg & Landreth, 1990). CCPT has been shown to be effective across multiple populations and multiple symptoms (Lin & Bratton, 2015; Post et al., 2019). Post et al. (2019) found that minoritized children responded better to CCPT as compared to directive play therapy modalities. Additionally, it has been shown to be effective in school-based settings, specifically on externalizing problems, internalizing problems, total problems, self-efficacy, academic, and other behaviors (Ray et al., 2015).

Cheng and Ray (2016) proposed that CCGPT address a child's social, emotional, and learning difficulties. CCGPT provides a safe space for children to develop coping behaviors, problem-solving skills, and self-expression skills (Cheng & Ray, 2016). School-based group play therapy has been suggested to be helpful with children who have experienced trauma (Shen, 2010) and Attention Deficit Hyperactivity Disorder (Reddy, 2010). Although there is currently a limited amount written on CCGPT, there are similarities between it and CCPT.

There are nonverbal and verbal skills used in CCPT that are also used in CCGPT to create a nonthreatening, appealing space for participants to feel safe in and connect with the MHP. Nonverbal skills include leaning forward/open, appearing interested, being relaxed/comfortable, speaking in a tone/expression that is congruent with child's affect, having the tone/expression congruent with the therapist's response, being succinct/interactive, and rate or responses (Ray, 2011). Verbal responses include tracking behavior, matching the child's affect, personalized responses, reflecting content, reflecting feeling, facilitating decision making/responsibility, esteem building/encouraging, and limit setting (Landreth, 2012). These skills are vital to creating a safe environment and strong therapeutic relationship. The nonverbal skills allow for participants to feel safe in the playroom and relate with the MHP, as well as increase the therapist's genuineness. The verbal skills are crucial to the MHP to accurately connect with and hear participants. In addition to these CCPT skills, facilitators must incorporate group skills such as linking to connect group members to each other.

There are special considerations when utilizing CCGPT. One consideration is that limit setting can be challenging for facilitators to implement. Although CCGPT and CCPT are different, there are similarities between the two with limit settings. Landreth (2012) stated, "limits are based on clear and definable criteria supported by a clearly thought-out rationale with furtherance of the therapeutic relationships in mind" (p. 261). Although this quote was written in reference to CCPT, it can be applied to CCGPT. In CCGPT things often move much more fast-paced than in individual therapy and the facilitator must be quick to set a limit if needed. It is up to the facilitators judgement when to set a limit, but they must keep in mind that the group participants safety is crucial. If a participant is risking the safety of the facilitators and group participants, they would need to step in and set a final choice limit that if the child chooses to continue the behavior they would choose to go back to class early. There is no specific rule on setting a final choice limit, it is up to the facilitator's judgement, but safety is the biggest consideration. Overall, safety of the students, group facilitator, and the room are used to determine what limits are necessary.

The group facilitators should also think about noise level. When completing a school-based CCGPT group, there is a chance the room being used is close to a classroom or another learning space in the school. This is where the MHPs can advocate for a more secluded room, or for sound machines to place outside of the room to limit potential distractions from the noise.

In order to complete a CCGPT group, there must be an appropriate space and toys for the groups. As stated previously, finding an appropriate space for play therapy in schools can be difficult. If you are conducting a CCGPT, it is crucial to have enough space for participants to move around freely. Landreth (2012) recommended a playroom size of 12 by 15 feet; however, that might be difficult in schools. As long as the space can be private, big enough for participants to move around, and have the appropriate toys in it; it can work.

Per Landreth (2012), the toys in the room facilitate the seven essentials in play therapy: 1) establishment of a positive self-relationship with the child, 2) expression of a wide range of feelings, 3) exploration of real-life experiences, 4) reality testing of limits, 5) development of a positive self-image, 6) development of self-understanding, and 7) opportunity to develop self-control. Additionally, he identified three categories of toys needed for a playroom: real-life toys, acting-out aggressive-release toys, and toys for creative expression and emotional release. It is recommended that the play therapist ensure they are acquiring culturally diverse toys/ materials for the playroom. Table 8.1 highlights a list of play therapy toys recommended for a playroom. Table 8.2 highlights a list toys recommended for a play therapy tote.

For there to be progress from CCGPT, it is recommended to complete six to eight sessions. It is important to schedule in flexibility to reach that six to eight session goal. There might be outside factors that could affect whether a group can meet in a given week, such as snow days, holidays, testing, and assemblies. There are multiple considerations when implementing a school-based CCGPT for students. In order to illustrate this, a case example of CCGPT with Marshallese-American kindergartners is provided. There is a large population of Marshallese-Americans where group relocation took place due to the United States relocating them from the Marshall Islands due to radiation contamination. There were no language barriers due to participants' first language being English.

Case Example

This section will discuss a school-based CCGPT group for Marshallese-American kindergartners at a school in the southern US. The group was funded by an external grant from the Association for Specialist in Group Work. The school counsellor worked with the authors to identify potential gaps to be addressed through group counseling. The school counselor identified that Marshallese-American students could benefit from a group experience to assist in their social, emotional, and academic development.

The school counselor had continuously advocated for play therapy in the school with administrators, and because of this, had full support for

Table 8.1 Playroom Toys and Materials

Play Therapy Toys for the Playroom		
Balls (large and small)	Egg cartons	Rubber knife
Band-aids	Empty fruit and vege-	Rubber snake, alligator
Barbie doll	table cans	Sandbox
Bendable doll family	Erasable nontoxic mar-	School bus
Blunt scissors	kers	Soap, brush, comb
Bobo (bop bag)	Flashlight	Spider and other insects
Broom, dustpan	Gumby	Sponge, towel
Building blocks	Hand puppets	Stove
Cereal boxes	Handcuffs	Stuffed animals
Chalkboard, chalk	Hats	Telephone
Colored chalk, eraser	Lone Ranger style mask	Tinker toys
Construction paper	Medical kit	Tissues
Crayons, pencils, paper	Medical mask	Tongue depressors,
Cymbals	Nursing bottle	popsicle sticks
Dart gun	Pacifier	Toy noise making gun
Dinosaurs, shark	Paints, easel, newsprint,	Toy soldiers and army
Dishes	brushes	equipment
Dishpan	Pitcher	Toy watch
Doll bed, clothes, blanket	Play Camera	Transparent tape, non-
Doll furniture	Play money and cash	toxic glue
Doll house	register	Truck, car, airplane,
Dolls, baby clothes	Pots, pans, silverware	tractor, boat, ambu-
Dress-up clothes	Pounding bench and	lance
Drum	hammer	Watercolor paints
	Puppet theater	Xylophone
	Purse and jewelry	Zoo animals and farm
	Rags and old towels	animal families
	Refrigerator	
	Rope	

Source: Adapted from *Play Therapy: The art of the Relationship (3rd Ed.)* (pp. 167–169), by G. L. Landreth, 2012, Routledge.

Table 8.2 Tote Bag Play Room Recommendations

Tote Bag Play Room Toys		
Aggressive hand puppet	Doll house	Popsicle sticks
Band-aids	Doll house furniture	Rubber knife
Bendable doll family	Handcuffs	Small airplane
Bendable gumby	Lone Ranger mask	Small car
Blunt scissors	Medical masks	Spoons
Costume jewelry	Nerf ball	Telephone
Cotton rope	Newsprint	Toy soldiers
Crayons	Nursing bottle	Transparent tape
Dart gun	Pipe cleaner	Two play dishes and
Doll	Playdough	cups

Source: Adapted from *Play Therapy: The art of the Relationship (3rd Ed.)* (pp. 166–167), by G. L. Landreth, 2012, Routledge.

individual and group play therapy. Additionally, the school counselor worked with the kindergarten teachers and explained the benefits of group play therapy for their students. The school counselor had teachers complete the Teacher-Child Rating Scale (TCRS) to use during the screening process. The kindergarten teachers provided feedback on the needs of their Marshallese-American students and this information was taken into consideration during the screening process.

Once potential students were identified the school counselor reached out to the student's guardians to obtain permission to participate in the group. After consent was provided, participants were screened with help from the school counselor and teachers and results of the TCRS. There were a total of eight Marshallese-American participants selected for groups. To keep the groups within a good ratio, they were split into two groups of four with two facilitators in each group. This section will focus on one group of four. There were a total of six 45-minute sessions for the group. The facilitators had decided to complete eight sessions over eight weeks with once a week 45-minute sessions; however, due to the COVID-19 pandemic, six sessions were completed.

The school counselor's advocacy for play therapy was beneficial for the group as there was a dedicated space provided for group play therapy. It was a private, quiet room, that was large enough for four participants and two facilitators and had all of the necessary toys as recommended by Landreth (2012). Additionally, based on Landreth's recommendations to have culturally inclusive toys, the school counselor and authors worked with the local Marshallese community group to identify appropriate toys for Marshallese-American children (see Table 8.3 for a list of specific toys

Table 8.3 Culturally Inclusive Toys

Marshallese Specific Toys
Dress-up (Hula Skirts)
Leis
Multicultural dolls*
Multicultural puppets*
Palm trees
Parrot puppet
Sand
Sandbox
Seashells
Shark puppet
Stuffed fish
Tropical play fruit
Ukulele
Wooden catamaran
Wooden drum

Note: *There were no Marshallese specific dolls, so the authors bought dolls and puppets that were most similar.

that were bought). Since there are limited options in schools for play therapy spaces, the meeting room did not follow all the recommendations for a playroom such as including a sink and bathroom, but it did have a window, that was covered with curtains and a carpeted floor.

This section will discuss one group's process throughout the six sessions. There were a total of four Marshallese-American kindergartners who participated in the group, with two males and two females between the ages of five and six. One facilitator was a Ph.D. student at the local university and the other was a school-counseling intern, both of whom had training and experience in CCPT. The four participant's pseudonyms were Robert, Jake, Marsha, and Jamie.

During the first group session participants did not engage in group play but were engaged in parallel play. Additionally, the children and facilitators were working on building trust with one another. The participants focused on using art materials and the sandbox but did not engage in play with other participants.

During the second session, three of the four participants played together, while Marsha played independently and kept an eye on the other participants. The three participants playing together played collaboratively in the sandbox and worked to get the facilitators' attention. Additionally, aggression was expressed through the use of the bop bag and throwing toys. Limits were set due to participants throwing toys and facilitators wanting to ensure everyone's safety.

All four participants began playing together in the third session. The children were engaged in a creative activity by coloring together and drawing similar pictures. Additionally, they worked on playing in the kitchen with food. Marsha began telling the other group participants that they needed to clean up and she took responsibility to ensure the room was clean before she left. The facilitators reflected that it was important for her to clean, but that she did not need to clean up before she left. Limits were set with Jamie as she did not want to leave when the group was done.

The fourth session also included all four participants playing together. Participants wanted the facilitators to shut their eyes, but a limit was set that our eyes had to stay open to ensure for safety, and this upset participants. Participants verbalized they were upset due to wanting to surprise the facilitators. The facilitators reflected participants feelings about being upset and how participants had planned a surprise for facilitators. The participants showed progress by expressing their frustration with facilitators through their words.

The fifth session began with all group participants playing together. Marsha began to appear less constricted in her play and less focused on the cleanliness of the room. The participants got into the sandbox and began dumping sand on themselves with no shoes on. Typically, the facilitators would set a limit on this, but a judgement call was made that this was an opportunity for group members, specifically Marsha, to be free and less concerned about making a mess.

In the last group therapy session, all of the participants played together. The children began to argue as to who would be playing with what toys but resolved the issue with their words. Facilitators reflected feelings during the argument and the participants were able to use their words and did not physically attack each other.

The group therapy facilitators did not have a chance to have a termination session due to the school closing because of COVID-19. The results from the post-TCRS showed an improvement for each participant. The group of four discussed in this section showed progress for all participants on the TCRS, thus providing support for MHPs to advocate with administrators on the efficacy of school-based play therapy. This data can be used with administrators moving forward to show the importance of implementing play therapy in schools.

Conclusion

This chapter discussed the considerations of implementing group play therapy in schools by Mental Health Professionals (MHPs). There are multiple roles that an MHP plays within the school, with their overall goal of helping students. Play therapy is the most appropriate way to address social emotional issues for children in elementary schools. Due to the disproportionate number of students to school-based MHPs, groups can be an efficient way to address multiple students' needs at once. The school-based MHP will need to advocate and educate school administrators and staff to use play therapy in schools. This chapter provided examples of how school-based MHPs can do this in schools. Child Centered Group Play Therapy (CCGPT) has been proposed as a developmentally appropriate play therapy group modality for children in elementary school and can be easily implemented in schools. Additionally, this chapter provided steps on how to implement a CCGPT, along with a case study of Marshallese-American kindergartners in a six-week CCGPT. School-based MHPs are encouraged to advocate for the use of play therapy in schools, specifically group play therapy to address the social emotional needs of their students.

References

Berg, C. R. & Landreth, G. L. (1990). *Group counseling: Concepts and procedures* (2nd ed.). Accelerated Development, Inc.

Cheng, Y. J. & Ray, D. C. (2016). Child-centered group play therapy: Impact on social emotional assets of kindergarten children. *The Journal for Specialists in Group Work*, 41(3), 209–237.

Center for Disease Control and Prevention. (2013). *Mental health surveillance among children – United States, 2005–2011*. www.cdc.gov/mmwr/preview/mmwrhtml/su6202a1.htm?s_cid=su6202a1_w.

Copeland, W., Wolke, D., Shanahan, L., & Costello, J. (2015). Adult functional outcomes of common childhood psychiatric problems: A prospective, longitudinal study. *JAMA Psychiatry*, 72(9), 892–899.

Department of Health and Human Services. (2000). *Report of the Surgeon General's conference on children's mental health: A national action agenda.* www.ncbi.nlm.nih.gov/books/NBK44233/.

Lambert, S. F., LeBlanc, M., Mullen, J. A., Ray, D., Baggerly, J., White, J., & Kaplan, D. (2007). Learning more about those who play in session: The national play therapy in counseling practices project (Phase I). *Journal of Counseling & Development*, 85(1), 42–46.

Landreth, G. L. (2012). *Play therapy: The art of the relationship.* Routledge.

Landreth, G. L., Ray, D. C., & Bratton, S. C. (2009). Play therapy in elementary schools. *Psychology in the Schools*, 46(3), 281–289.

Lin, Y. W. & Bratton, S. C. (2015). A meta-analytic review of child-centered play therapy approaches. *Journal of Counseling & Development*, 93(1), 45–58.

O'Connell, M. E., Boat, T., & Warner, K. E. (Eds.) (2009). *Preventing mental, emotional, and behavioral disorders among young people: Progress and possibilities.* The National Academic Press.

Perryman, K. L. (2010). Guidelines for incorporating play therapy in the schools. In Drewes, A. A. & Schaefer, C. E. (Eds.), *School-based play therapy* (2nd ed. pp. 61–86). John Wiley & Sons, Inc.

Perryman, K. L. (2016). Play therapy in schools. In K. J. O'Connor, C. E. Schaefer, & L. D. Braverman (Eds.), *Handbook of play therapy* (2nd ed. pp. 485–504). John Wiley & Sons, Inc.

Post, P. B., Phipps, C. B., Camp, A. C., & Grybush, A. L. (2019). Effectiveness of child-centered play therapy among marginalized children. *International Journal of Play Therapy*, 28(2), 88–97.

Ray, D. C. (2010). Challenges and barriers to implementing play therapy in schools. In Drewes, A. A. & Schaefer, C. E. (Eds.), *School-based play therapy* (2nd ed., pp. 87–106). John Wiley & Sons, Inc.

Ray, D. (2011). *Advanced play therapy: Essential conditions, knowledge, and skills for child practice.* Routledge.

Ray, D. C. & McCullough, R. (2016). *Evidence-based practice statement: Play therapy.* www.a4pt.org/?page=EvidenceBased.

Ray, D. C., Armstrong, S. A., Balkin, R. S., & Jayne, K. M. (2015). Child-centered play therapy in the schools: Review and meta-analysis. *Psychology in the Schools*, 52(2), 107–123.

Reddy, L. A. (2010). Group play interventions for children with Attention Deficit/Hyperactivity Disorder. In Drewes, A. A. & Schaefer, C. E. (Eds.), *School-based play therapy* (2nd ed., pp. 307–329). John Wiley & Sons, Inc.

Shen, Y. J. (2010). Trauma focused group play therapy in schools. In Drewes, A. A. & Schaefer, C. E. (Eds.), *School-based play therapy* (2nd ed., pp. 237–256). John Wiley & Sons, Inc.

Simon, A. E., Pastor, P. N., Reuben, C. A., Huang, L. A., & Goldstrom, I. D. (2015). Use of mental health services by children ages six to 11 with emotional or behavioral difficulties. *Psychiatric Services*, 66(9), 930–937.

Sweeney, D. S. (2011). Group play therapy. In Schaefer, C. E. (Eds.), *Group play therapy: Foundations of play therapy* (pp. 227–252), John Wiley & Sons, Inc.

Trice-Black, S., Bailey, C. L., & Kiper-Reiechel, M. E. (2013). Play therapy in schools. *Professional School Counseling*, 16(5), 303–312.

U.S. Department of Health and Human Services Administration for Children and Families Office of Planning, Research and Evaluation. (2010). *Head Start impact study final report.* www.acf.hhs.gov/sites/default/files/opre/hs_impact_study_final.pdf.

Yalom, I. & Leszcz, M. (2005). *The theory and practice of group psychotherapy* (5th ed.). Basic Books.

Yee, T., Ceballos, P., & Swan, A. (2019). Examining the trends of play therapy articles: A 10 year content analysis. *International Journal of Play Therapy*, 28(4), 250–260.

9 Group Play in Hospitals

Child Life Playrooms

Joan Turner and Jessika Boles

Certified Child Life Specialists (CCLSs) are healthcare professionals who use play-based techniques to meet the developmental and coping needs of children and families navigating healthcare encounters (Association of Child Life Professionals, 2020; Turner, 2018). Recognizing healthcare events as challenges to children's typical participation in their families and communities, CCLSs integrate six domains of theory and practice (see Figure 9.1) as they provide goal-oriented play opportunities in healthcare settings; specifically, their work combines:

> ...1) an individualized approach to care, 2) a focus on cultivating resilience, 3) cognizance of the developmental contexts in which children and families live and grow, and 4) consideration for the impacts of past and present trauma, [thereby] CCLSs 5) establish and develop therapeutic relationships by 6) capitalizing on the expansive utility of play.
>
> (Boles et al., 2020; p. 3)

Although this emphasis on play resonates with underpinnings of the play therapist profession, CCLSs articulate their interventions as a form of *therapeutic play* – not therapy – meaning that play is used to help children meet normative developmental and coping goals rather than address clinical pathologies or psychological disruptions (Turner, 2018; Williams et al., 2019). The opportunities for therapeutic play that CCLSs offer to young people in hospitals, specifically in designated playroom spaces, invite children of all ages to step away from the pressures of the healthcare environment into a space and experience designed with their needs and interests in mind.

Hospital Playrooms: Moving from Then to Now

In 1910, the first hospital-based play program was started at Massachusetts General Hospital (Turner & Brown, 2014). As national interests in child health and welfare grew throughout the 20th century, additional

DOI: 10.4324/9781003094531-9

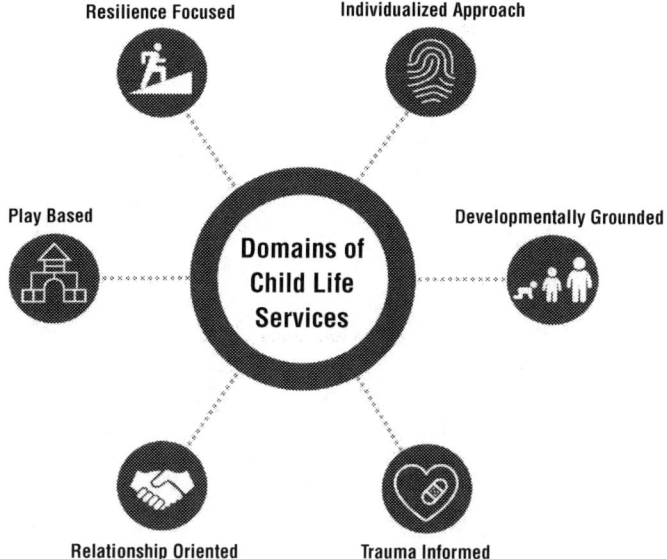

Figure 9.1 The Six Domains of Child Life Practice
Source: Figure courtesy of the Association of Child Life Professionals

children's hospitals established formal play programs to meet the needs of pediatric patients and mitigate the long-term behavioral impacts of hospitalization. Yet, it was not until 1965 that six founding women gathered, along with 40 leading professionals from 23 facilities across the United States and Canada, to formalize the work of play specialists – soon to become CCLSs – across North America (Turner & Brown, 2014). The perspectives on play held by this fledgling Association for the Care of Children in Hospitals (ACCH) were largely informed by the work and advocacy of child life pioneers Emma Plank, Mary McLeod Brooks, and Barbara Jean Seabury. These early child life professionals led the charge for play and educational programming, viewing play as an inarguable right for children and youth coping with illness and injury. Often described at that time as "play ladies", these hospital-based play specialists soon came together to solidify their professional identity as child life specialists, subsequently forming the Child Life Council (CLC) in 1982 (renamed as the Association of Child Life Professionals in 2017).

Empirically and academically, CCLSs are largely recognized for their provision of evidence-based stress-point preparation (Boles, 2016; Boles, 2018a; Boles et al., 2020; Grissom et al., 2016) and procedural support interventions (Boles, 2013; Boles, 2018b; Boles et al., 2020; Burns-Nader et al., 2017; Moore et al., 2015) for children undergoing painful or invasive procedures. Since the seminal works of Visintainer and Wolfer (1975), and the landmark research of Thompson and Stanford (1981), CCLSs have carried on the legacy of using age-appropriate communication, educational tools, and both directed and non-directed play opportunities to help children anticipate, express their feelings about, and cope with the stresses of medical care.

What is lesser espoused about the child life field, however, is its continued commitment to group play provision. In the eyes of hospitalized children and their families, the trusting relationships and supportive presences that CCLSs establish through play are most valued; these relationships are the primary tools by which CCLSs help children understand and manage their feelings about their healthcare encounters (Boles et al., 2020). Play – whether offered individually or in group sessions – affords each child, no matter the limitations of their illness and injury, an opportunity to feel safe, secure, and in control of their thoughts, feelings, and healthcare experiences (Williams et al., 2019). Even as contemporary healthcare practices and philosophies evolve to stress the more "clinical" sides of medical and psychosocial care, it is the opportunities for self-expression, empowerment, and exploration that CCLSs have facilitated and advocated for since the field's inception.

In the eyes of CCLSs trained and working in the field prior to the new millennium, the prominence of child-life-supervised group play appears to have declined, particularly in hospital playrooms. During the late 1980s, child life programming had a prominent presence in and focus on the physical playroom space available in most pediatric hospitals and units. In addition to group play and free play opportunities, early hospital playrooms often included group mealtimes. Additionally, some play programs featured scheduled or structured programming for young people from morning through the evening – as well as weekends. The playroom in this era was characterized by a constant presence of child life specialists coming and going as they escorted children from the wards and introduced them to the playroom environment. Work time for these professionals was devoted to the building of relationships with young people through engagement in group play (therapeutic or diversional), building rapport, and facilitating assessment in a safe space. In essence, child life was synonymous with both bedside play and the playrooms in the hospital. Subsequently, new expectations for the role of the child life specialist emerged and began to extend their clinical reach beyond dedicated play spaces. The resulting sense of a separation between play and clinical roles is documented to arise when the professional and peer-reviewed literature is examined.

Current Research on Playrooms in Healthcare Settings

Play remains a crux of child life practice in healthcare and community settings today, although systematic evaluation of scholarly and professional publications reveals a lack of research regarding play-based interventions

– especially compared to the mountain of evidence documenting the effects of psychological preparation and procedural support by child life specialists (Boles et al., 2020; Boles et al., 2021; Turner & Boles, 2020). More specifically, examinations of the contemporary scope of child life research in peer-reviewed journals, and the Association of Child Life Professionals' publication, *Child Life Focus*, have been completed (Turner & Boles, 2020; Boles et al., 2021). Primarily, the frequency of peer-reviewed journal articles related to play-based child life interventions enjoys a sizeable increase through the 1990s and early 2000s, but then decreases after 2007 (Boles et al., 2021). Although there is no single factor that this shift can be attributed to, it is interesting to notice that published articles related to psychological preparation and coping support interventions during medical procedures rise just as articles centered around play interventions begin to decline.

On the other hand, as recently as 2020, a renewed interest in group play is seen in Jones and colleagues' evaluation of a group medical play intervention and children's self-reported fear and anxiety in the pre-operative waiting room. Based on structured observations and interviews with five-to ten-year-old children scheduled for surgery, it was found that a child-life-specialist-facilitated group medical play intervention was not only clinically feasible and acceptable to patients and families (Grissim et al., 2020), but the intervention was also associated with a statistically significant decrease in child anxiety per the modified-Yale Preoperative Anxiety Scale (m-YPAS) (Kain et al., 1997). Perhaps these emerging efforts are indicative of future directions for child life research, resisting the individualist focus of many of today's procedure-focused interventions, and returning to the group-based, socialization-driven play opportunities that generated a child life profession and accompanying line of inquiry.

What is evident in these scoping reviews and emerging studies is a limited, although perhaps shifting, presence of play intervention research and descriptions, both in *Child Life Focus* and peer-reviewed journals. However, in its humble beginnings, group play was at the forefront of child life programs in healthcare settings. It is this historical foundation, and lack of current investigation, that led us to conduct a narrative inquiry study on the group play practices and perceptions of CCLSs. Once IRB approval was received, a sample of 35 CCLSs working in the United States and Canada participated in narrative interviews or focus groups about their group play programs and approaches to play provision in healthcare settings. Ranging from two to more than 35 years of clinical experience, these participants reinforced the importance of group play, particularly in designated play spaces (playroom, teen lounge), and articulated the benefits of group play for young people in hospital, their families, child life programs, and healthcare institutions. Thus, although empirical evaluations of group play programs led by CCLSs are currently limited, these participants validated that group play is very much alive and vibrant in healthcare settings across North America and that there is value to continued investment in play programs for hospitalized children and their families.

Features of Group Play Programs in Healthcare Settings

Each hospital playroom program – and even each playgroup interaction – is uniquely shaped by a variety of environmental, developmental, and contextual factors that must be navigated by children, families, and child life professionals to bring group play opportunities to fruition. Given the intentional nature of child life group play interventions in children's healthcare settings, it is important to note that the individual child's needs and characteristics will factor strongly into the features of group play in a playroom setting.

Impact of Hospitalization

Certified Child Life Specialists and those involved in group play programs must continually assess the impacts of the healthcare environment and treatment regimen on the child's ability to participate in play opportunities. Elements as straightforward as a child's attachment to an IV pole for antibiotic therapy, or as complex as the toddler living with tracheostomy and ventilator dependence, must be foreseen, and planned for, in order to create a safe – and impactful – play experience for children of all needs and abilities in hospitals. Thus, CCLSs must consider elements of medical and psychological safety, adequately accessible space and medical resources, and adaptable equipment, materials, and staffing to help children participate in the ways that are possible and meaningful for them.

As medical complexity increases, the availability of parents/caregivers at the child's bedside can also impact on the structure and availability of group play programs in healthcare settings. Parents and other legal or familiar caregivers can be valuable supports not only during their child's overall hospital stay, but also in helping their child access play groups and helping staff get to know their child's play needs and preferences. However, noting that this is not always possible for families juggling a wide variety of social and familial responsibilities in and beyond the hospital, parental presence and availability is a factor that CCLSs consider when attempting to design group play programs that are as accessible and equitable as possible.

Intentionality

Once patient and family needs are assessed and anticipated, and institutional resources are garnered, group play opportunities then require an investment of time, energy, and expertise into each stage of the group process – from planning to implementation and finally evaluation. Although much of this work is done by CCLSs assigned to specific patient care units, clinics, wards, or physical playroom spaces, these efforts often require partnership with additional staff such as hospital volunteers, child life assistants or activity coordinators, or even medical staff in the cases of those children with complex medical needs or specialized equipment. Each step of playgroup planning must be done with intentional consideration of children's abilities, developmental needs and concerns, unique interests and play preferences, patient and family goals, and the dynamics of group formation and supervision. In some healthcare centers, these developmental capabilities or limitations have even resulted in play spaces stratified by age group, mobility level, or isolation requirements. These features then, in turn, shape the child life specialist's ability to plan and provide group activities.

Outcomes of Child Life Playroom Programming

In attempting to present group play led by CCLSs in healthcare playroom settings, it is important to note that there is no one-size-fits-all approach to these interventions and programs. However, through engagement with institutional resources, and investments of time, energy, and staffing into planning and providing group play programs, it is possible to engender a host of outcomes for hospitalized children, their family members, and the professionals and institutions that serve them. These outcomes can range from in-the-moment benefits such as positive engagement and a sense of control in the unpredictable healthcare environment, to long-term effects such as the creation of family-centered memories and establishment of coping mechanisms that will serve the child throughout their lifespan.

Although empirical evidence on the outcomes of group play for children, families, and programs in healthcare settings is currently limited, CCLSs describe a large array of observed benefits for children of all developmental levels and cultural backgrounds. First and foremost, group play opportunities can restore a sense of normalcy that is often lost during a hospitalization or healthcare encounter; group play in this setting can help the child access familiar activities and play equipment that will help them feel comfortable in this new and stressful environment. Additionally, they can exercise or regain the developmental skills they have relied on and will continue to need after their healthcare experiences. Furthermore, play groups create opportunities to meet and find support in peers who can relate to the child's feelings and experiences in this space, and generate positive relationships with staff that will continue to be involved in their care. This exposure to supportive others can help children learn about their diagnosis, treatment, and even techniques for coping with the stress generated by these events.

Play also affords the child an opportunity to make choices and feel a sense of control in an environment in which autonomy is often limited by illness and treatment. Through play, they can find the confidence to share their feelings, ask questions, or express the meanings they are constructing about their healthcare experience. These feelings of empowerment and engagement can refine and strengthen the child's coping skills both within the walls of the playroom, as well as the confines of their hospital room or even the procedure room. When opportunities for medical play or art with medical themes are purposefully integrated into group play programming, this non-threatening exposure to medical equipment and processes can scaffold the child's developing health literacy (Turner & Dempsey, 2017). Children can feel more prepared for – and able to – manage their participation in medical procedures and treatments (Boles, 2018b; Grissom et al., 2016).

Planning and Providing Playroom Play and Activities

Group play opportunities in hospital settings require intentional planning on the part of the CCLS and other responsible professionals. This preparation should not only involve planning the materials and features of the group play offering, but also attending to the availability, interests, and abilities of the patients that will potentially participate. Often for CCLSs, this is a dynamic process (Turner & Fralic, 2009) by which interventions and activities are generated based on known patient and family needs and readily adaptable for young people of any condition.

Given the limitations of funding and space that many group play programs experience in healthcare settings, preparing a group play activity may begin by inventorying and procuring needed supplies, or by considering clinical assessments of patient and family needs to identify a goal for the group play experience. These assessments may consider which patients are medically able to leave their rooms, the level of staff involvement or accompaniment needed for the patient's safety, and any potential overlaps in age groups, diagnoses, or play interests that can be used to help individuals connect with one another during the play group. As these plans are formed, CCLSs work to foresee any adaptations that may need to be made, to ensure that the appropriate materials and space will be available.

CCLSs design group play opportunities in healthcare settings around the developmental, coping, and psychosocial needs of the young people and families they serve. Based on the information gathered in their assessments of individual patients and unit-based needs, they may create singular or recurrent play groups that can help children and families meet developmental milestones, express their thoughts and feelings, and harness the coping skills needed to manage those thoughts and feelings adaptively. In some programs, the underlying goals of group times are determined largely by the CCLS, whereas others involve collaboration with social work, rehabilitative and speech therapies, or creative arts therapies. In healthcare settings focused on injuries to the brain or spine, or those treating children with complex healthcare needs, this collaboration is essential given the functional and developmental goals of the child's overall care plan.

It is important to note that the same play group goals can be accomplished in a variety of play-based ways. Examples of group play activities in healthcare settings range not only with respect to the goals of the experience, but also the level of structure (or freedom) the activity presents, the length and type of social interactions needed to participate in the activity, and whether the activity is more adult-directed or child-directed. What appears to be most important in providing high-quality group play experiences is the goodness-of-fit between the individual participants, the carefully facilitated group interactions, and the features of the play experience.

Certified Child Life Specialists, some of whom hold dual credentialing as Certified Therapeutic Recreation Specialists, describe group play opportunities based on their identified goals for children and families including: 1) developmental/functional, 2) therapeutic/expressive, 3) socialization/connection, 4) normalization/recreation, and 5) medical play (see Figure 9.2). Developmental or functional play groups are centered around achieving or strengthening specific skills or abilities in the wake of illness, injury, or long-term hospitalization. For example, at a pediatric rehabilitation hospital, an adaptive version of soccer using foam pool noodles, extra shoes and leg braces, and a ball is regularly provided to help children with limited mobility strengthen their upper body musculature and improve hand-eye coordination – while engaging with a local professional soccer club. Therapeutic or expressive play groups are focused on helping young people identify and express their thoughts and feelings related to the features or impacts of their illness or injury. One CCLS described a teen group in collaboration with the spiritual care department that brings teens together to discuss the difficult aspects of their care that they may not feel comfortable sharing with others – which at times has culminated in a group art project or contribution to the hospital environment.

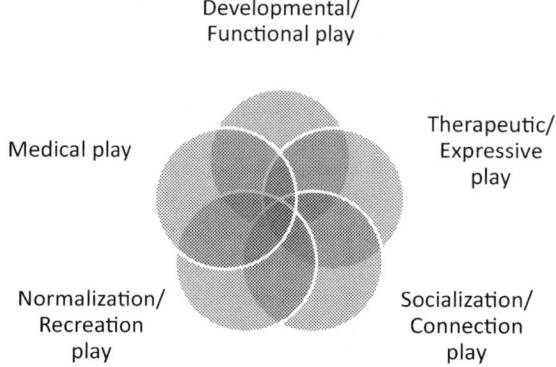

Figure 9.2 Taxonomy of Group Play Opportunities in Healthcare Settings
Source: Figure courtesy of Joan Turner and Jessika Boles

Groups focused on socialization and connection are designed to help children and family members with similar circumstances or conditions encounter one another, in the hopes that such a meeting might spur an ongoing relationship by which all parties can find social support in one another. Recreational play groups, or those focused on normalization, are engineered to help bring familiar elements of play into the unfamiliar environment of the healthcare setting; these groups translate beloved activities and play interests from home into the hospital playroom to reduce anxiety and assist the child in finding normalcy amidst change. Finally, medical play groups use real or pretend medical equipment in either adult-directed or child-directed ways as a means of helping children learn about, become familiar with, and exercise control over their health-care experience. These activities can range from "teddy bear clinics" to syringe painting, each of which incorporates medical supplies in a way that allows children and youth to encounter, rehearse, and master elements of their care in a playful way.

Case Example: Teen Lounge in a Rehabilitation Hospital

The CCLS working in a rehabilitation hospital with adolescents and young adults providing group programming in a teen lounge with long-term patients is highlighted. The teen lounge Child Life Specialist is just one member of the health care team responsible for providing interventions to groups of young people as they freely engage in recreational, diversional, and therapeutic play and activities in a space designated specifically for their needs. Traumatic experiences can be a common factor across this patient population with traumatic brain injuries, spinal cord injuries, motor vehicle accidents, and gunshot injuries. Pain, grief, and ambiguous loss in addition to long-term separation from family, friends, and community represent a sample of concerns that arise as individuals convalesce and rehabilitate while in-patients. Clara, a Playroom CCLS, put it this way, "teens are already going through [so much] in general development and life that it is incredibly challenging at that stage. And then to be in the hospital, it is even then more stressful. And then, to be in a children's hospital where so much is oriented around younger kids… [there are] multiple layers of challenge and ways that teens can feel unheard or unseen, so we serve a very valuable role in being able to advocate for teens."

Some patients come to the teen lounge with some form of medical equipment whether it be a wheelchair, IV pole, or other assistive device. However, the space is considered a "neutral" area with no medication delivery or invasive health care assessments and treatments allowed. The teen lounge is designed to accommodate groups of patients whose size and requisite medical equipment necessitates a larger space which is extended when access to outdoor areas is scheduled. Play and project materials are accessible to teens and young adults in a play space designed to accommodate independent play and small and large group interactions at tables of various sizes and shapes, in family style sitting areas, and in open spaces allowing for sitting on the floor or participating in limited movement-based play and activities. Some advanced materials, such as digital cameras, tablets, desk top computers, and video editing equipment, or expensive art materials, are kept in locked cupboards for use during interventions developed with specific outcomes in mind.

The teen lounge is quite different from a playroom in terms of how it is structured. There are more open-ended offerings in the form of a project or a design experience. Arts-based or science-based materials are offered in addition to interaction-based games such as Uno. Multiple planned activities are available daily, but on a flexible schedule as the CCLS will respond to individual needs, interests, and requests, as well as ideas that arise through peer interactions. Planning is done in response to which long-term patients familiar to the program will be attending and through communication with them to determine interests and engagement. Invitations are relayed to patients who often come and go as they desire.

Programming in the teen lounge is about making the play and activities individualized and patient-focused, never directive: "The most meaningful times I have seen that happen is when children are imitating and then they are feeding off of each other so they develop something that each of them individually may not have thought of (Clara)." Examples of group activities include collaborative journaling, spin art, murals, and film making. Examples of group activities involving inter-professional collaboration include extending school projects into the teen lounge, movement activities supported by physical and occupational therapists, and artists-in-residence programs. Clara described the "Fun Friday" collaborative outdoor event at her facility, "The teens do therapy but in a way that's more directive or fun or just to end the week in a really positive or exciting way for kids – where they look forward to it. We'll do a scavenger hunt or some sort of project: this week we're going to do tie-dye outside."

Thus, it is evident that CCLSs approach hospital-based group play activities with an interest in creating trusting relationships with young people through interaction and responsivity to observed needs and interests. The core of the child life teen lounge programming is creating a foundation of connection and community and building relationships with young people and between the young people.

Returning to the Value of Play

Although play is a child's most innate tool for learning, communication, and connection, it is important not to underestimate the value of skilled play group facilitation – especially in stressful contexts such as healthcare settings. Certified Child Life Specialists facilitating group play experiences speak to the careful balance that must be struck between attending to the needs of each individual child in the group while also being cognizant of and responding to group dynamics. In a hospital playroom, group inter-actions are simultaneously happening at several levels: between parents/caregivers and other staff present in the room, and the direct interactions children are engaging in with one another. Thus, supervising a group play experience requires attention to a variety of concurrent processes, between patients, parents/caregivers, and staff, while maintaining a focus on the identified goals of group.

Although the value of group play opportunities may appear most rele-vant for pediatric patients themselves, it is important to acknowledge the host of outcomes that parents/caregivers, siblings, and staff can experience. Just as the child can benefit from the social connections that take place in the playroom, so too can parents and siblings as they connect with others that can relate to their thoughts and feelings. Beyond an increase in social support, parents/caregivers and siblings can also benefit from the oppor-tunity to see their ill or injured child partake in fun and enjoyable activ-ities amid stress and uncertainty. In the playroom, families can create positive memories during their healthcare experience, feel a sense of release from the stresses of illness and injury, and bond in familiar and meaningful ways. Seeing their child laugh, make choices, and act as they would at home or at school can give families positive interactions with their child that they may not otherwise get to experience in the healthcare environment.

Group play programs are also an excellent opportunity to demonstrate the power of play in children's lives, and the direct impact of child life services on children and their families. Such programs can help to advo-cate for, secure funding for, or grow CCLS positions and group play offerings so that more patients and families can benefit from the restora-tive power of play, developmentally appropriate education, and family support. Simultaneously, there is also great value in these programs for other medical and psychosocial healthcare team members as they can observe children in their natural element – play. The greater result, though, may be in the coping benefits that come from staff being able to see their patients happy, engaged, and able to experience a sense of wonder and joy even during a stressful healthcare encounter.

References

Association of Child Life Professionals. (2020, October 31). *What is a Certified Child Life Specialist?*www.childlife.org/the-child-life-profession.

Boles, J. C. (2013). Speaking up for children undergoing procedures: The ONE VOICE approach. *Pediatric Nursing*, 39(5), 257–259.

Boles, J. C. (2016). Preparing children and their families for procedures or surgery. *Pediatric Nursing*, 42(3), 36–39.

Boles, J. C. (2018a). Preparing children for healthcare encounters. In J. Rollins, C. Mahan, & R. Bolig (Eds.), *Meeting children's psychosocial needs across the healthcare continuum* (2nd ed., pp. 43–78). Austin, TX: Pro-Ed, Inc. www.proe dinc.com/Products/14266/meeting-childrens-psychosocial-needs-across-the-healthcare-continuumsecond-edition.aspx.

Boles, J. C. (2018b). The powerful practice of distraction. *Pediatric Nursing*, 44(5), 247–253.

Boles, J., Turner, J., Rights, J. D., & Lu, R. (2021). Empirical evolution of child life 1998–2017: A scoping review of child life content in published research. *Journal of Child Life* 2(1), 4–14.

Boles, J. C., Fraser, C., Bennett, K., Jones, M., Dunbar, J., Woodburn, A., Gill, M., Duplechain, A., Munn, E., & Hoskins, K. (2020, March 1). *The value of Certified Child Life Specialists: Direct and downstream optimization of pediatric patient and family outcomes (Full report)*. www.childlife.org/docs/default-source/the-child-life-profession/value-of-cclss-full-report.pdf?sfvrsn=5e238d4d_2.

Burns-Nader, S., Joe, L., & Pinion, K. (2017). Computer tablet distraction reduces pain and anxiety in pediatric burn patients undergoing hydrotherapy: A randomized trial. *Burns*, 43(6), 1203–1211. doi:10.1016/j.burns.2017.02.015.

Grissim, L., Kirkendell, M., Jones, M., & Boles, J. (2020). Medical play and children's self-reported fear in the pre-operative setting. *The Journal of Child Life*, 1(2), 7–15.

Grissom, S., Boles, J. C., Bailey, K. C., Cantrell, K., Kennedy, A., Sykes, A., & Mandrell, B. N. (2016). Play-based procedural support and preparation intervention for cranial radiation. *Supportive Care in Cancer*, 24(6), 2241–2427. doi:10.1007/s00520-015-3040-y.

Jones, M., Kirkendall, M., Grissim, L., & Boles, J. C. (2020). Effect of a group medical play intervention on children's pre-operative anxiety. *Accepted for publication in Journal of Pediatric Health Care*. Published ahead of print at: www.jpedhc.org/article/S0891-5245(20)30211-X/abstract.

Kain, Z. N., Mayes, L. C., Cicchetti, D. V., Bagnall, A. L., Finley, J. D., & Hofstadter, M. B. (1997). The Yale Preoperative Anxiety Scale: How does it compare with a "gold standard"? *Anesthesia & Analgesia*, 85(4), 783–788. doi:10.1097/00000539-199710000-00012.

Moore, E. R., Bennett, K. L., Dietrich, M. S., & Wells, N. (2015). The effect of directed medical play on young children's pain and distress during burn wound care. *Journal of Pediatric Health Care*, 29(3), 265–273. doi:10.1016/j.pedhc.2014.12.006.

Thompson, R. H. & Stanford, G. (1981). *Child life in hospitals: Theory and practice.* Chicago, IL: Charles C. Thomas. www.ccthomas.com/details.cfm?P_ISBN13=9780398044565.

Turner, J. (2018). Theoretical foundations of Child Life. In Richard H.Thompson (Ed.), *Handbook of child life* (2nd ed., pp. 34–54). Chicago, IL: Charles C. Thomas. www.ccthomas.com/details.cfm?P_ISBN13=9780398092122.

Turner, J. & Boles, J. C. (2020). A content analysis of professional literature in the Association of Child Life Professionals' focus: 1999–2019. *The Journal of Child Life: Psychosocial Theory and Practice*, 1(1), 7–16.

Turner, J. & Brown, C. (2014). *The pips of child life.* Dubuque, IA: Kendall Hunt. https://he.kendallhunt.com/product/pips-child-life-early-play-programs-hospitals.

Turner, J. & Dempsey, V. (2017). Preschooler's health care play: Children demonstrating their health literacy. In L. Rubin *Medical play therapy and child life: Clinical interventions for children and adolescents* (pp. 19–37). Routledge. doi:10.4324/9781315527857.

Turner, J. C. & Fralic, J. (2009). Making explicit the implicit: Child life specialists talk about their assessment process. *Child & Youth Care Forum*, 38(1), 39–54.

Visintainer, M. A. & Wolfer, J. A. (1975). Psychological preparation for surgical pediatric patients: The effect on children's and parents' stress responses and adjustment. *Pediatrics*, 56(2), 187–202.

Williams, N. A., Ben Brik, A., Petkus, J. M., & Clark, H. (2019). Importance of play for young children facing illness and hospitalization: Rationale, opportunities, and a case study illustration. *Early Child Development and Care*, 191(1), 58–67. doi:10.1080/03004430.2019.1601088.

10 Group Play Therapy in Therapeutic Residential Care

David A. Crenshaw and Domonique Garrett

Overview and Perspective

Therapeutic Residential Care (TRC), is a high level, intensive, and expensive model of care, which serves youth who suffer from complex trauma. In 2021, the Families First Act takes effect, which may create significant changes in this treatment model. The Families First Act is an initiative of the Federal Government, designed to keep children and adolescents out of congregate care facilities and in their families and home communities whenever possible. Only youth with the most severe disorders will be eligible for referral to TRC. The authors share the spirit and philosophy of this legislative thrust which is to treat children within their homes or as close to home and family as possible although it remains to be seen what challenges accompany this major initiative.

Given the severity and multiple sources of trauma suffered by the typical youth placed in TRC, conducting group play therapy can be both an exciting and daunting challenge. Clinical experience in leading groups in TRC includes preschool play therapy groups (Crenshaw et al., 2015), psychoeducation groups within the Sanctuary Model (Bloom, 2013), special focus groups such a grief and loss (Crenshaw, 2005, 2008, 2014b), DBT groups, social skill groups, sibling or family groups (Crenshaw et al., 2015; Crenshaw et al., 2018), family play therapy (Crenshaw, 2014a, Crenshaw et al., 2016; Gil et al., 2017), assertion and anger management groups (Badau et al., 2005; Crenshaw & Foreacre, 2001), and bonding/attachment groups for high-risk young mothers and their babies (Carnes & Crenshaw, 2015).

Each age, developmental level, type of group, or group focus presents its own unique challenges and therapeutic benefits. Some of the above listed groups share the goal of teaching specific skills or imparting important knowledge such as the DBT, psychoeducation, social skills, assertion, and anger management groups. Other groups are focused on relational and attachment issues such as sibling groups and parent-child attachment/ bonding; while special focus groups are purpose driven and goal-structured (see Sweeney et al., 2014 for a comprehensive description of different types of therapeutic play groups).

DOI: 10.4324/9781003094531-10

Brief Overview of Group Play Therapy in Therapeutic Residential Care

In TRC, typical therapeutic challenges are intensified by the extent of the trauma suffered by the typical youth referred for out-of-home group congregate care (Wilcox, 2014). In TRC programs, youth assessed on the adverse childhood questionnaire have averaged a 5.8 adverse childhood experiences (ACEs) score (any score 4 and above is considered clinically significant). In addition, by the time youth arrive for TRC, the typical youth is disenchanted with most forms of therapy and reluctant to commit to any outpatient model (Crenshaw et al., 2020; Wilcox, 2014). Group therapy in TRC, including group play therapy, may be more appealing to some youth than individual sessions. In either form of therapy, adolescents often feel their vulnerabilities are exposed but some would prefer that exposure to take place among their peers rather than alone with an adult.

There are challenges in TRC groups due to the high level of prior trauma exposure. This can create issues in establishing safety due to the high frequency of triggering trauma memories, and youth at different stages of readiness to confront upsetting topics. In TRC groups, it is extremely hard to establish safety. Even in groups whose purpose is psychoeducation, triggering can easily occur resulting in explosive emotional reactions that frighten both the youth and their peers. Another obstacle for the group leader is that group members can be on different social/emotional developmental levels and at different stages of readiness to confront traumatic material and memories. This has been especially taxing in specific focus groups like grief and loss or sexual abuse survivor groups. One answer to this dilemma is that play allows for self-pacing even in a group context. An example of this occurred in the Attachment/Bonding Play Group for young at-risk mothers and their babies. All the young mothers had suffered extensive trauma. While other mothers in the group were able to master their anxiety sooner which allowed them to get on the floor and engage in playful interactions with their babies, one unusually traumatized mother who had suffered chronic and ritualistic abuse took a whole year to accomplish the same step (Carnes & Crenshaw, 2015).

To discover the elements of success within TRC groups, experienced clinicians* and group facilitators were surveyed by the authors. The surveyed clinicians have been successful in leading groups with youth in group congregate care. The authors asked what these clinicians found to be keys to success and the following points were emphasized:

1 Buy In: Youth are made aware from the beginning of the sessions that attending group is an important part of the program and they are expected to attend. Incentives, including treats, are sometimes provided to reinforce their participation.
2 Structure: Recognizing the presence of trauma symptoms and acknowledging the role trauma responses play in residential centers means we

must carefully design groups to maintain the upmost safety. This is especially important in the early stages before group cohesion is achieved. Negotiating group agreements with teens helps to create safety, enhance trust, and formulates a container of the space. Agreements serve as co-created guidelines to clearly inform how to operate inside the structure with respect and responsibility. This allows each group member to have a stake in the group environment and provides opportunity for each member to hold one another accountable. Organizing the room in a circle enhances accountability and helps the facilitator be alert to indictors of traumatic stress.

3   Clear Expectations: The kinds of behaviors considered constructive and conversely disruptive are explained when initially meeting with the youth. The purpose of the group is shared to gauge interest and willingness to participate. This process allows the group to take ownership. When disruptions arise, modeling acceptance with a range of people's expressions and listening attentively to the words expressed lets the group members know they are understood, heard, and validated. Active listening skills included focusing, reframing, asking clarifying questions, and acknowledging feelings. This may require the facilitator to move away from the agenda to best meet the needs of the group.

4   Consistency: Unplanned (illness, crisis, AWOLs) and planned events (family visits, medical appointments, etc.) play havoc with weekly scheduled meetings. When consistency breaks down it devalues the importance of the group. This is true whether the inconsistency is on the part of the youth or the staff leaders.

5   Planning: It is helpful to have a topical outline for each week of group prepared with multiple hands-on activities youth chose from each session. Topical outlines help the facilitator guide the discussion and keep it focused. Allowing the group to choose from a menu of activities engages the group from a youth-centered approach. The planned activities enable group buy-in and participation. Providing youth with a menu of activities to choose from rather than articulating what activity they wish to do reduces verbal demands.

6   Collaboration: Asking the youth for their input and ideas about what they would like to do in session and what they hope they will gain, helps the group leader to foster investment. The member's feedback and voice are valued. It contributes to the unique structure of the group and strengthens their commitment to show up for one another. The group facilitator establishes a caring environment by responding to group needs and requests in a timely manner allowing the facilitator to learn more about the participants.

7   Empowerment Based: A strength-based approach based on resilience research promotes a sense of power from within by supporting the youth's self-determination and autonomy. Active listening and believing

in the youth's ability to take care of themselves and articulate what they need strengthens autonomy. In addition, empowerment activities are chosen to help youth regulate their trauma and learn about "mental tools" they can take away with them.

8　Use of Metaphor: During adolescence, youth are developing the capacity to apply language to their emotions. Given the complex history of residential youth, often these emotions are too overwhelming to speak out loud. Adolescents in TRC, however, can express strong emotions safely through creative arts, video tapes, and poetry. For example, discussing interactions between characters in a movie scene, including feelings and motives, can be less intimidating than identifying their own personal feelings. In these moments, the clinician leading the group challenges youth to explore their sense of self, to feel rather than avoid or distract, and to acknowledge their ability to hold discomfort while remaining safely within the windows of affect tolerance.

9　Staff Support: In TRC, the encouragement of staff in the program, especially youth counselors in the cottage group, can make the difference between success and failure. When staff take the time to build a caring and consistent relationship with the youth, this can form some of the most positive and supportive environments a youth will experience. This is important as youth frequently take their cues from their house staff who, depending on whether they value the group, can be encouraging and supportive of a youth's participation, or at the other extreme, discouraging, or indifferent. When staff are willing and invited to participate in the group sessions, this communicates to the youth the space is safe, builds courage within the youth to speak up, and enhances the staff to youth relationship through creating meaningful conversation with one another.

10　Cultural Competence: The ability to look through different lenses and respectfully see various viewpoints is essential to cultural competence. To run a culturally relevant group, it is helpful to consider how culture and oppression affect the experiences of group members. An understanding of how cultural groups have different experiences within dominant mainstream systems becomes pertinent to addressing the challenges minority groups may face. Facilitators should remain mindful of power dynamics and remember they are not the leaders of the group, the youth are.

11　Small Moments Matter: Trust is built upon small, simple moments over time. Remembering significant group interactions, special events, birthdays, or specific individual needs represents genuine care for each group member. In these groups, the therapist takes time and care to repair relationships. When working with youth who have had their boundaries and trust shattered, the responsibility as caring therapists is to take interactions with youth seriously and allow young individuals the ability to heal wounded spaces within themselves.

*The authors wish to thank the following experienced clinicians and group facilitators for their valued input: Kara Cannelli, Courtney Doyle, Amy Elmanakhly, Lori Stella, RaeAnn Tompkins, and Amy Westberg.

Research and Theory on Group Play Therapy in Therapeutic Residential Care

There is power in group therapy. In group play therapy, there is not only power but magic. Group play therapy has many benefits in TRC. It allows the adolescents a safe place to explore and express their thoughts and feelings through play. It is extremely important for the practitioner to create an environment that is welcoming to them. By creating a positive environment, youth can comfortably add their input (Cooper, 2000) which builds self-esteem and leads to a positive group experience. When working with youth in a play therapy group, practitioners must take into consideration social and cultural experiences. This enables us to not rush to assumptions, judgements, or generalizations (O'Connor, 2005) about behaviors of children and adolescents during group play therapy.

On the best days, youth in TRC can behave in unpredictable and volatile ways, consistent with the high level of trauma and correlating dysregulation that can occur. Examples of this include adolescents running out of the room, confronting peers or the group leader, yelling loudly and sometimes adopting combative body stances, and even physical fights can happen although not frequently. The group facilitator must be prepared for a range of possibilities. Defusing tense situations as quickly as possible are fundamental tools and crucial for maintaining safety. DBT skills (Rathus et al., 2014) especially in distress tolerance, emotional regulation, and interpersonal effectiveness are important in keeping affect within windows of affect tolerance (Siegel, 2020). DBT skills are taught and practiced in both individual and group therapy sessions in TRC. One way to regulate the emotional temperature in the room is for the leader to shift focus when discussions are triggering group members and the safety of the group is threatened. Shifting to DBT skills, especially distress tolerance skills, practicing self-soothing, improving the moment, and/or distraction skills may help to manage the group within the windows of affect tolerance.

Play Therapy Group Case Study and Intervention

In the following section, the authors will first share with you an example of group play therapy in keeping with a Child Centered Play Therapy approach. We will also share two therapist directed play therapy interventions consisting of *Puppet Scripts* to facilitate sharing of vulnerable feelings of fear, sadness, and worry. When engaging in playful interventions, the therapist can help to allay anxiety and threatening feelings using metaphor and masking symbols.

Group Example

This vignette will focus on a play therapy group with four young boys ages 7–8 years old who resided in an RTC. These young children became the therapist's (DG) first play therapy group. The boys shared similar struggles in their homes, in the classroom, and within the residential treatment setting. Their teachers and guardians shared concerns regarding their emotional and behavioral outbursts. The children would not sit still, follow directions, and would become dysregulated during structured classroom time. The initial session was very memorable, for many reasons. The four boys arrived at the play therapist's office all at once. A staff member ushered the four boys into the office and quickly closed the door. For the first five minutes the four little boys stared at the play therapist in silence. One little boy, Matt, was the first to speak. He said in matter-of-fact voice, "We are here because we're bad." The other three boys quickly agreed, nodding their heads. The second little boy, David, turned and knocked the doll house and doll house figurines to the ground. He then turned and looked at the therapist, who simply said, "You knocked that down." John, the third little boy then said, "You are supposed to yell and punish him." The therapist responded, "He will not get in trouble in here for knocking down the doll house." As if he would like to test that theory, the fourth boy, Mark, went and knocked over the Duplo blocks. Once the boys realized the therapist would not yell or punish them, the four boys proceeded to knock all the toys off the shelves and push them to the center of the floor with pleasure.

After the boys finished with this play, they were invited to sit at the table with the therapist and his co-facilitator – an anxious squirrel puppet named Sam. Sam the Squirrel explained to the boys that in the beginning of each group we would pick feelings cards and "check in" with our feelings. On the table, feelings cards were placed face up. The boys were invited to pick the feeling(s) they had felt that day. Sam then picked a feelings card. Sam was used to express how sad he gets when adults yell at him. One at a time the boys began to express their feelings about past and current stressors. Matt said he felt scared when his mom used to forget to pick him up from school. David expressed his sadness about a recent fire in his family's home. Mark stated he felt "a big worry" that his family would never find a new home and John expressed missing his dad who recently went to jail. After validating these worries, Sam the Squirrel taught the group members about "checking in", the group structure and format, and at the end of the group, Sam would teach a new coping skill. To the surprise of the therapist, the boys sat, listened, and even asked Sam questions.

Matt, who was quickly taking on a leadership role in the group, asked "What's a coping skill?" Sam, being the anxious squirrel he is, became extremely nervous and worried that he would not answer the question correctly. John quickly comforted him and suggested "Mr. C. can tell the group." The boys eagerly moved to learning the deep breathing coping skill through blowing bubbles. They were directed to take large breaths and blow it out slowly to form a bubble. After practicing bubble blowing, the boys were invited to play with anything they wanted in the playroom. Each boy got up from the table and selected a few toys. Matt selected blocks and moved to a corner of the room. He turned his back to the group and began building. John selected cars and the track mat. He sat in the middle of the room and began to play. David selected the doll house and its figures; he too found a space and turned his back to his peers. Mark simply sat at the table and colored. The therapist engaged in child-centered play therapy, using tracking with each boy and their individual play until the end of group that day.

The combination of directive and non-directive play led to a positive group experience for each client. It aided in transforming the group space into a safe and inviting place where the boys could express their feelings and learn new skills.

Play Therapy: Group Structured Intervention

In play therapy groups with frequent turnover in membership, therapists typically structure the groups starting with warm-up activities that include teaching calm and self-soothing activities, followed by a period of free play, and ending with a closing activity of singing a song (to increase a sense of community) and saying goodbye. Sometimes the degree of structure in TRC, especially in younger groups, aligns with a more structured play therapy intervention such as Puppet Scripts that set the stage for safely exploring feelings further within metaphor as illustrated below:

*Puppet Script # 1 – Adventures of Frog and Turtle (created by 1st author)**

Rationale: vulnerable emotions such as fear, sadness, and worry are hard to acknowledge particularly in the presence of peers. This structured puppet scenario provides not only a playful context which allays anxiety (Schaefer et al., 2014) but utilizing the third person puppet characters provide masking symbols (Sarnoff, 2002) to keep the threatening emotion at a safe symbolic distance. Enabling expression of the threatening emotions through the puppets is a step toward mastery of the worries and fears.

Intervention

Two puppets, Freddy Frog (therapist) and Tommy Turtle (co-therapist), engage in a dialogue about overcoming fears. The group facilitator teaches the puppets about emotions and feelings, utilizing the third person (puppets) to help minimize the vulnerable experience for the group members, as talking directly about fears may be threatening to some children. The therapist begins by introducing the topic. "*Today we are going to call on two of our puppet friends to talk about fears. We want to introduce you to two of our favorite puppets, Freddy Frog and Tommy Turtle. They are going to tell you about some of their adventures together.*" The therapist and co-therapist then lend their voices to the puppets to continue the playful discussion.

FREDDY FROG: "So, you see, when our friendship started out Tommy was a scaredy cat. He feared everything. He feared shots, loud noises, other animals, especially alligators, but now because of my help, he is one brave Turtle."

TOMMY TURTLE: "Freddy is right I used to fear all kinds of things but not anymore. Even though I did not want to go, Freddy talked me into going with him on adventures that scared me such as going up in a hot air balloon, and another time we crossed the desert, and still another time we went up in a spaceship. I was scared at first, but then I discovered that facing my fears little by little helped me to overcome them with the help of my friend Freddy. I cannot believe it but now all my friends think I am brave."

The therapist then invites each group member to pick a puppet. Speaking to the chosen puppets, the therapist addresses each of the puppets with the question: "Are there any fears that you are hoping to overcome? Maybe not a big one, perhaps a little one? Frog and Turtle are here to listen and to help." The therapist then invites each child to be the voice of their chosen puppet. The therapist encourages each child to voice any fears of their puppet they are willing to share with the group. The children take turns naming the fears of their puppets. If the child's puppet can admit to a fear, it is best to stay in metaphor and call on Frog (voice of therapist) and Turtle (voice of co-therapist) to respond first by listening and normalizing the fear and then to make some tentative suggestions that will help the puppet to gradual mastery of the fear. Suggestions from other puppets can be elicited before moving on to the fears of the next puppet.

Sample Dialogue

CHILD'S PUPPET: "I am a little scared of the water. I do not know how to swim."

TOMMY TURTLE: "I felt the same way before I entered the water at first. My mom kept me in the shallow water at first, teaching me just to play and have fun. Little by little, she encouraged me to go further out but slowly until I was comfortable. Now swimming is one of my favorite things to do. I spend a lot of my time in the water and it is so much fun."

FREDDY FROG: "Tommy's mother taught him to be playful and enjoy the water, is there someone who helps you feel safe that could help teach you to enjoy the water just like Tommy, a little at a time? The main thing is to take your time and learn to play in and enjoy the water."

Puppet Script # 2 – Sadness, Anxiety, and Grief in the Pandemic

The lives of children and youth in foster care are replete with loss and trauma. The COVID-19 pandemic has added additional stress, isolation, and separation from loved ones including no in-person visits or only technological visits taking place through remote video sessions. This has correlated to an increase in anxiety, depression, and frustration as well as anger.

Intervention

This intervention was developed to help the residents cope with the challenges COVID-19 has brought to the RTC. In this group, the puppets have a conversation about their thoughts and feelings regarding sadness and frustration. One child at a time in the group is invited to choose a puppet. For example, the child chooses a puppet called Sarah and the therapist picks a puppet called Ben.

BEN: "Is it okay Sarah if we talk about sadness today?"

BEN: "Many times, lately, I feel sad because it is hard for me to see my family. How about for you Sarah?"

SARAH: "Same here. Sometimes I break down and cry after my video family visits because I just want them to hug me."

BEN: "I cry sometimes too, but usually in my room alone. You are brave Sarah to cry in front of others. I wish boys could do that but boys are taught they are not supposed to cry. Boys are afraid other kids will call them a big sissy."

SARAH: "I do not cry often but when I do other kids and staff do their best to cheer me up."

BEN: "I guess because boys do not show it, nobody knows when they are upset. Sometimes boys think that others just don't care. But they are so good at hiding their tears others don't realize they are upset."

SARAH: "One of the hardest things for me is that nobody knows when this virus will end."

BEN: "You are so right Sarah. None of us know and that makes it so hard. I am wondering about the rest of you, what has been the hardest part for each of you coping with this crummy virus? I think it is okay to be mad about this virus and all the ways it has changed our world."

SARAH: "Do any of you know someone who is sick from the virus?"

BEN: "Whom do you worry about the most?"

BEN: "I want to hear about everyone's best coping strategy during a tough time like this."

SARAH: "Great idea! Would someone make a list of all the coping skills we share?"

BEN: "Sometimes, coping with difficult situations make us stronger. Can anybody give an example of how you learned something valuable during this crisis?"

*The first author wishes to thank Elizabeth Kjellstrand Hartwig for her encouragement and review of these puppet scripts.

Conclusion

Group play therapy in a therapeutic residential care setting presents a host of challenges to test the mettle of the therapist. Groups of all kinds in TRC can be taxing to the group and therapist alike due to the level of trauma exposure among the youth which frequently leads to a traumatic triggering response within the members when sensitive topics arise. Planning for such groups is hindered due to various factors including the reality that each group participant may be at different levels of readiness to approach the material that is the focus of the group. Consequently, groups frequently require considerable thought and sensitivity to the diverse needs of the group and emotionally charged trauma triggers for each member. Group play therapy has inherent advantages because of the healing powers of play and the inherent support of group membership and the sense of community play can bring to the therapeutic process. As group members share their feelings through play together, it normalizes their experiences, emotions, symptoms and reduces the sense of shame and isolation that many residents of RTC experience. Complex traumatic experiences are often experienced as stigmatizing.

Play therapists know that playful interactions allay anxiety and enable our youth to face what otherwise might be overwhelming. Therapeutic play enables mastery at the pace that is tolerable for each youth (Schaefer et al., 2014). While challenging, group play therapy in therapeutic residential care offers many rewarding and gratifying moments for the play therapist seeing growth unfold in both the individuals and group.

References

Badau, K. & Esquivel, G. B. (2005). Group therapy for adolescents with anger problems. In L. Gallo-Lopez & C. E. Schaefer (Eds.), *Play therapy with adolescents* (pp. 239–266). Jason Aronson.

Bloom, S. (2013). *Creating sanctuary: Toward the evolution of sane societies* (2nd ed.). Routledge.

Carnes, S. & Crenshaw, D. A. (2015). The dance of resilience and attachment in high-risk mother-infant relationships. In D. A. Crenshaw, R. Brooks, & S.

Goldstein (Eds.), *Play therapy interventions to enhance resilience* (pp. 194–217). Guilford Press.

Cooper, R. J. (2000). The impact of child abuse on children's play: A conceptual model. *Occupational Therapy International, 7,* 259–276.

Crenshaw, D. (2005). New clinical tools to treat childhood traumatic grief. *Omega: Journal of Studies of Death and Dying,* 51, 235–251.

Crenshaw, D. A. (2008). Overview of grief therapy with adolescents. In K. Doka (Ed.), *Living with grief: Children and adolescents* (pp. 217–232). Hospice Foundation of America Press.

Crenshaw, D. A. (2014a). Play therapy approaches to attachment issues. In C. A. Malchiodi & D. A. Crenshaw (Eds.), *Creative arts and play therapy approaches for attachment problems* (pp. 19–32). Guilford.

Crenshaw, D. A. (2014b). Counseling adolescents. In K. J. Doka & A. S. Tucci (Eds.), *Helping adolescents cope with loss* (pp. 323–340). Hospice Foundation of America Press.

Crenshaw, D. A. & Cannelli, K. (2020). Reflections on "stealth therapy" in Therapeutic Residential Care. *Residential Treatment for Children & Youth,* 37(3), 244–264.

Crenshaw, D. & Foreacre, C. (2001). Play therapy in residential treatment. In A. Drewes, L. Carey & C. Schaefer (Eds.), *School-based play therapy* (pp. 139–162). John Wiley & Sons.

Crenshaw, D. A. & Gil, E. (2016). Family drawing in couple and family therapy. In J. L. Lebow*et al.* (Eds.), *Encyclopedia of couple and family therapy.* https://doi.org/10.1007/978-3-319-15877-8_561-1.

Crenshaw, D. A. & Kelly, J. E. (2018). The use of puppets in psychodynamic child therapy. In A. A. Drewes & C. E. Schaeffer (Eds.), *Puppet play therapy: A practical guidebook* (pp. 86–97). Routledge.

Crenshaw, D. A. & Tillman, K. S. (2015). Trauma narratives with children in foster care: Individual and group play therapy. In D. A. Crenshaw & A. L. Stewart (Eds.), *Play therapy: A comprehensive guide to theory and practice* (pp. 262–275). Guilford Press.

Dickens, C. (1859). *A tale of two cities.* Reprinted by International Collectors Library. Garden City, NY.

Gil, E. & Crenshaw, D. A. (2017). Play in couple and family therapy. In J.L. Lebow*et al.* (Eds.), *Encyclopedia of couple and family therapy.* https://doi.org/10.1007/978-3-319-15877-8_546-1.

O'Connor, K. (2005). Addressing diversity issues in play therapy. *Professional Psychology: Research and Practice,* 36(5), 566–573.

Rathus, J. H. & Miller, A. L. (2014). *DBT skills manual for adolescents.* Guilford.

Sarnoff, C. A. (2002). *Symbols in structure and function, Volume 2: Symbols in psychotherapy.* Xlibris.

Schaefer, C. E. & Drewes, A. A. (Eds.) (2014). *The therapeutic powers of play: 20 core agents of change.* Wiley.

Siegel, D. (2020). *The developing mind: How relationships and the brain interact to shape who we are* (3rd ed.). Guilford.

Sweeney, D. S., Baggerly, J. N., & Ray, D. C. (2014). *Group play therapy: A dynamic approach.* Routledge.

Wilcox, P. D. (2014). *Trauma-Informed treatment: The restorative approach* (2nd printing). NEARI Press.

11 Group Play Therapy in Outpatient Settings

Clair Mellenthin

Group play therapy can be a powerful agent of change for children. Group therapy is effective for children throughout the developmental span of childhood, including adolescence (Bratton, et. al, 2009; Chinekesh et. al, 2013; Morshed et. al, 2019; Perryman et. al, 2015). According to the most recent National Mental Health Services Survey (2018), the majority of mental health services take place in outpatient settings (Substance Abuse and Mental Health Services Administration, 2018). This necessitates outpatient-based play therapists to utilize individual, family, and group play therapy to effectively treat a wide variety of emotional and behavioral issues in children.

Group play therapy is a powerful treatment modality to help children navigate the challenges they face, as well as celebrate new beginnings, new chapters, and a new sense of *self* throughout the healing process. So often in today's world children experience increasing isolation, loneliness, and feelings of helplessness. Their window for connection with other same-age peers during school is limited as recess and play time is shortened or may be taken away all together (Perryman, 2016). During the global COVID-19 pandemic, many children have been quarantined at home, with online learning and online social interactions taking the place of in-person engagement. Group play therapy may be more important than ever as our world comes out from its cocoon of seclusion.

Brief Overview

Landreth (1991) wrote:

> Group play therapy is a dynamic approach which holds great promise for improving, expanding, and enhancing the play therapy relationship to meet the existing needs of children. In this relationship, children learn from each other, encourage each other, support each other, work out difficulties, share in pain and joy, discover what it is like to help each other, and discover that they are capable of giving as well as receiving help.
>
> (p. xii)

DOI: 10.4324/9781003094531-11

Given the nature of outpatient work, whether it is brief short-term therapy or long-term therapy, there is more flexibility and ability to engage in a creative, therapeutic process. Due to the large number of children engaging in therapeutic services in outpatient settings, facilitating group play therapy is a way to help clients find a sense of connection to others, as well as be able to treat similarly diagnosed children in larger numbers.

When starting a new play therapy group, it is helpful to have an identified cluster of child clients who are currently receiving individual and/or family therapy services at the same outpatient therapy center. This allows for an immediate group cohort rather than attempting to start a group for the community at large where there may be a perceived need but not the clientele in place to begin. Creating groups in this way is particularly helpful for those in private practice or smaller community mental health centers without a specific identified client population. It is also important to have a play space large enough to comfortably accommodate a number of children at one time. Be aware that group play therapy can be loud – full of giggles, laughing, talking, and movement. When working in outpatient therapy spaces, being mindful about when and where to hold the group play therapy sessions is important, this might include consulting with and informing fellow therapists in the clinic and neighbors in the office building. It is often helpful to inform the other tenants of the office building where the group will be meeting, as well as ask them if there are preferred days or times to hold group play therapy so that it does not impact their businesses. Most neighboring businesses have been welcoming of the information and their frustration decreases when they understand the reason behind the increased noise and why so many children are coming in at one time.

Group play therapy may consist of as few as two children at a time to facilitating groups with large numbers of children attending. This author recommends starting with a base of three children at a minimum, as this helps to promote group cohesion, as well as the ability for the group to maintain itself whether the group is short-term or an open-ended group. It is the experience of this author that both short-term and open-ended styles of group play therapy have been shown to be successful in outpatient therapy services. It is encouraged to have a co-facilitator when there are groups larger than six children. This helps to contain the chaos, encourage personal connection and relationship with each child, as well as help with direction and engagement. Having a co-facilitator involved also offers a different therapeutic perspective, as well as engagement strategies which can be beneficial to the therapeutic process.

Depending on the age of the group members or treatment issue, it may or may not be important to have same gendered peers in the group membership (Sweeney & Homeyer, 1991). Being mindful of both the developmental needs of the age of the child, as well as the treatment issues being addressed, can help in the decision-making process. Keeping the chronological as well as emotional ages consistent in the group members is important when engaging in group play therapy, as this helps to promote group continuity, sharing, and connection (Bratton et al., 2009; Kulic et al., 2001). Employing screening measures to ensure that the group members' coping skills complement each other, have a similar level of interest, and capacity to form peer relationships is also an important undertaking (Bratton et al., 2009). It is also critical to assess and screen for the client's background history to prevent exposing group members to inappropriate information and behaviors (2009). In addition, parental consent is required for group work to commence.

Facilitating group play therapy can be a richly rewarding experience – and takes a lot of patience, flexibility, and adaptability to be successful. Due to the nature of working with several different children simultaneously, it is critical for the facilitator to have strong boundaries, behavior modification training, and a good sense of humor. Using humor to diffuse aggression, non-compliance, and disinterest can go a long way in developing rapport and a therapeutic relationship (Mellenthin, 2020). Incorporating play-based regulation and co-regulation activities at the start and ending of each group session can be beneficial for both the facilitator as well as the clients (Hudspeth & Matthews, 2016). This helps to keep the clients focused, as well as engaged in the therapeutic group process. In addition, this provides the child with a consistent closing activity they can look forward to and understand that the time is up, and it is time to say goodbye. Clapping games, rhythmic activities, dancing, special handshakes, and upbeat music are great ways to facilitate engagement at the beginning of the group play therapy session. This helps to "warm up" the brain and body together, as well as provides the children an opportunity to play and engage together (2016, p. 595). Ending activities that "cool down" the brain and physical activity are just as important (2016, p. 595). Finger painting, bubble breathing, guided imagery, and yoga stretches are fun ways to help the children connect to one another as well as calm their bodies down at the end of the group activity.

Establishing group rules and having the child participants create and agree to the group rules can help to reign in some of the chaos that group play therapy can bring to the office (Ray, 2011). Other than the rule that people are not for hurting, rules should be set by the children and not the therapist. This helps to create a sense of connection and empowerment between the group members from the beginning. This author will bring a large posterboard to the group and invite the children to write down their decided rules together, the poster is then hung on the wall for all to see. Allowing the children to name their group and to create a mascot together using expressive arts materials is another fun, playful way to begin building bridges of connection and communication. This is often done in the first group session.

The nature of the group structure varies depending upon the theoretical orientation and group model chosen. This author engages in an integrative, prescriptive model of play therapy, incorporating various tenets of play therapy theories and interventions. By utilizing an integrative approach, the play therapist is able to identify specific needs of each group member, as well as the group needs as a whole and create or employ therapeutic interventions to meet the treatment needs. Regardless of the theoretical model chosen, allowing for autonomy and group interaction is important in group play therapy. Interventions should be playful and inclusive, empowering the child clients to take the lead and engage with one another.

Research

Research has shown that group play therapy is effective at treating a myriad of emotional and behavioral issues typically seen in outpatient settings including diagnoses of Oppositional Defiant Disorder (Dillman Taylor et al., 2019; Meany-Walen et al., 2014; Morshed et al., 2019), Autism Spectrum Disorder (Grant & Turner-Bumberry, 2020), limited social skills (Blalock et al., 2019), issues of grief and loss (Webb, 2010), as well as families experiencing divorce and separation (Rich et al., 2007). For a large number of child clients seen in outpatient therapy services, a formal mental health diagnosis may not be warranted. These children experience difficulties in navigating social situations, regulating impulses, and lack confidence and feelings of self-worth. For the purposes of this chapter, attention will be focused on group play therapy with elementary age children experiencing socio-emotional difficulties.

Swank et al. (2017) found that in the elementary school years, children learn either adaptive or maladaptive foundational social skills and emotional responses that will help contribute to future success or long-term struggles. The development of attention skills and prosocial relational skills help children as they grow and mature. A child's development of healthy socio-emotional competencies is related to their ability to succeed and thrive in life (Blalock et al., 2019). For a child struggling to develop these important life skills, they often experience interpersonal challenges across environments. They may engage in externalizing behaviors such as low frustration tolerance, aggression, hyperactivity, low impulse control, defiance, and experience poor relationships with peers and family members. This makes for a difficult life experience, with constant friction between parent and child, teacher and child, as well as between peers and child. Without therapeutic intervention, these children are at risk for developing long-term developmental challenges including school suspensions, poor academic performance, teenage pregnancy, drug abuse, and future antisocial behaviors (Swank et al., 2017; Dillman Taylor et al., 2019).

Merrell (2011) identified social and emotional assets as

> a set of adaptive characteristics that are important for success at school, with peers, and in the outside world. They include facets such as friendship skills, empathy, interpersonal skills, social support, problem solving,

emotional competence, social maturity, self-concept, self-management, social independence, cognitive strategies, and resilience.

(p. 3)

Through group play therapy, children with socio-emotional difficulties have the opportunity to interact with peers and adults in a much more positive manner. They are able to learn how to develop these needed positive social and emotional assets as they are able to try on new personalities or ways of managing emotions. They may find a place of acceptance and unconditional positive regard by a kind, helpful adult. They may realize that they are not alone in their problems as they meet with other children with similar experiences or emotional challenges. It is through these experiences within the group process that creates an environment where children can improve social skills, learn adaptive behaviors, increase self-regulation, improve cognitive flexibility, and develop empathy (Meany-Walen & Kottman, 2019).

Within the group play therapy experience, children learn friendship-making skills as well as learn to accept responsibility for their actions. They may have an opportunity to be in a positive leadership position within the group experience. It also provides space where they can learn to make and keep friends, manage emotions appropriately, and learn prosocial skills. For many children who struggle across environments including school, home, family, and peers, it is a rare occurrence to feel positive about themselves and be engaged in these positive experiences. These experiences are necessary to build their self-esteem and positive sense of self-worth.

Research has shown that children with disruptive behaviors who participate in group play therapy demonstrate improvements in behavioral, emotional, and social learning (Morshed et al., 2019; Woolf, 2011). As they experience positive growth and personal development, children learn to apply their newfound skills and knowledge to outside relationships which positively impacts their home, school, and peer relationships (Dillman Taylor et al., 2019; Kottman, 2011; Meany-Walen et al., 2015; Sweeney et al., 2014). As the child's worldview slowly begins to shift and change, and their ability to recognize triggers and learn ways to control for these triggers, they begin to feel more confident in navigating their world. Through the group experience children are able to feel connected to and a part of something positive. For many children it is in group play therapy where they feel accepted for the first time; for who they are, and as they are. As Landreth (2016) noted, "A child will change when they feel like they don't have to change, meaning that once a child can feel accepted *as* they are, for *who* they are, there is room to make changes and therapeutic progress will commence."

This is not to say that group play therapy experiences are always positive and easy to facilitate, particularly within this subgroup of socio-emotional disturbances. The group facilitator may be faced with a challenging environment and challenging participants. The play therapist needs to be able to accept there will be chaos, and the "inevitability of human contact over which the therapist has no control" (Ray, 2011, p. 183). Some of this human contact may include poor physical boundaries, aggression, hyperactivity, and dysregulation. Feeling comfortable with and knowing that there are situations and experiences that you may not have total control over is important for the facilitator to understand when holding group therapy. The play therapist needs to be flexible and adaptable in their therapeutic approach and with the children involved. The play therapist may need to change the day's planned activities to meet the emotional or behavioral needs of the group on that particular day and be willing to hold firm boundaries and expectations simultaneously. This is another reason why having a co-facilitator involved is important, particularly when working with a group where aggressive or challenging behaviors are present and part of the treatment focus. This allows for one facilitator to continue working with the group, while the other works to help calm or regulate a dysregulated or disinterested child. By working in conjunction with one another, the therapeutic goal of bringing the dysregulated child back into the group activity/process is achieved.

Yalom (1995) believed that group play therapy creates opportunities for children to authentically act as they would in the real world. With the buffer of the therapeutic relationship in place, children can experience more adaptive responses to the world around them. It is through the interpersonal and intrapersonal processes of group play therapy where children can learn new ways of being with another, as well as with themselves.

Group Example/Intervention

Katie, Alex, James, Marco, and Vanessa, all age 9, were referred to outpatient individual play therapy services. Exhibited difficulties included: lack of social skills, anger management, and emotional outbursts taking place at home and in school. It was assessed that these five children could benefit from participation in group play therapy, with the therapeutic goals identified as 1) improve social skills, 2) learn healthy coping skills, 3) develop appropriate expression of emotions, and 4) make and keep friendships. The therapist met with each child's parents to discuss how group therapy would be beneficial, as well as assess the appropriateness of each child's participation based upon their background history. The therapist then met with each individual child to assess their level of functioning, develop positive therapeutic rapport, and invite their participation to the group process.

On the first day of group, the therapist could hear the children before she saw them in the waiting room. One was yelling loudly at his mother, protesting his involvement in the group. Another was crying and saying she did not feel safe being there. Another parent could be heard giving a consequence and threatening to take their child home if they did not sit still. A scuffling was taking place between siblings and they began wrestling on the floor. To say it felt chaotic on this first meeting would be an understatement. Due to the level of dysregulation present before the group had even started, the therapist decided to walk into the waiting room and engage in a clapping game with all of the children and their parents before taking them into the group play room. She began by clapping very softly and asking those who could hear her to join in the rhythmic game. One by one, each person in the waiting room was able to engage and participate in the clapping. As this happened, regulation occurred, and a calmness resumed in the waiting room.

As the children regulated their bodies as well as their mood, the therapist led them into the group play therapy room, still engaging in a rhythmic clapping game. Once inside, the therapist asked the children to sit in a large circle and introduced herself. After explaining confidentiality, she placed a large posterboard in the middle of the group and asked them to think of the "rules" they would like to create. The children were able to problem solve together and create the group norms and rules. They decided that 1) everyone had to wear shoes so there would be no stinky feet; 2) no pushing or hurting people; 3) no yelling or swearing; 4) take turns speaking; and 5) the therapist would bring a treat to every group if they were good.

In each group, the therapist engaged in prescriptive play therapy interventions, tailoring the group activities to meet the needs of the group as whole, as well as each individual child. In this particular group, many of the children had experienced bullying in one form or another. Some had been victims of extensive bullying by their peers at school, while others had engaged in bullying behaviors. During one group, the children were shown the Pixar^{TM} short *For the Birds*. They were then asked to identify the challenges each of the different birds faced, as well as what happens when the group began bullying one of the birds. After exploring and processing this aspect of the video, the children were asked which bird they most identified with and was given clay to create a bird that best represented them. They were then able to share with one another their clay creations, as well as what it felt like to be a bird who bullied, was bullied, or was a bystander. Through this activity, the children learned the meaning of empathy, compassion, and standing up for themselves and others. Alex shared that he had been bullied in the past and shared his experience of feeling humiliated and alone in his experience. Marco was quick to jump in and attempt to comfort him by offering to beat up the bullies for him. Katie was able to process feeling helpless when she had witnessed bullying take place to one of her friends and had stayed silent during the experiences. She shared that she had felt too scared that she would be the next bullying victim if she spoke up. As the children began sharing their individual experiences, they were able to listen, and join with one another.

In the ensuing weeks, the children began developing closer relationships together. The therapist could hear them gather in the waiting room and within a few weeks, she could hear the excited greetings as they gathered together in the waiting room. During week four, which is typically the halfway point and the "storming phase" (Tuckman, 1965) of group work, it is common for intragroup conflict to occur. This group was no exception to this as at the beginning of group, James came into the group room visibly upset and angry. He grabbed a toy that Vanessa had been playing with and threw it across the room away from her. When she protested and told him to stop, he stomped over to the corner of the room and began kicking the wall. The therapist walked over to him and remarked that it appeared he was feeling frustrated and wanted to show the group how big his feelings felt inside. She handed him a squishy ball and redirected the kicking by offering something he could throw against the wall without damaging it. James was surprised that he was not in trouble and looked suspiciously at the therapist, stating, "You're just trying to get me in more trouble!" The therapist answered, "James, in here, you don't get into trouble. I can see that there are some big feelings inside of you, and all of your feelings are important and matter to me. I wonder if you can show me or use your words to tell me about these big feelings instead of kicking the wall or teasing your friend. Here, I will show you" and the therapist proceeded to throw the ball against the wall exclaiming, "I feel so mad when someone cuts me off when I am driving!" She handed the ball to James, motioning him to throw the ball. James gingerly took the ball from the therapist and looked for permission one more time before throwing the ball exclaiming, "My teacher is the worst person in the entire universe!" By now, all of the other children were quiet and watching this exchange take place. One by one, each of the children took a turn throwing the ball and stating something they either did not like or felt mad about. The therapist had planned a different activity for the week's group but could quickly see that there needed to be cathartic play instead. She quickly brought in some Splat!^{TM} balls and gave one to each child. They spent the rest of the group throwing the balls against the wall as they identified different emotions and experiences where they had felt that feeling. As the group regained a sense of cohesion and joining, the emotions shifted, and as a group they were able to choose different emotions to talk about, focus on, and process. James in particular had a significant shift in his mood and behavior, as he was able to release pent-up emotions and process his "no good, very bad day" with his friends. At the end of the group session, James walked up to Vanessa and apologized for his actions. She graciously accepted his apology and they walked out together to meet their parents.

On the last day of the group, the therapist asked the children to create a sandtray together that represented their therapeutic journey. The children were able to process their emotions and experiences together, as they created the sandtray, each adding in their chosen miniatures. As the group ended, the therapist handed each of the children a small paper bag that held a small item that represented each of the different week's topics and a coping skill the children had learned. She gave each child a small toy butterfly to represent their growth and learning as they walked out the door and said goodbye to one another.

Conclusion

Sweeney and Homeyer's (1991) advice rings true in contemporary times, "Group play therapy should facilitate the establishment of a therapeutic relationship, the expression of emotions, and the development of insight, and it should provide opportunities for reality testing and for expressing feelings and needs in more acceptable ways" (p. 13). Group work is a fun, challenging, and exciting method of engaging in play therapy in your clinical practice. Group play therapy in an outpatient setting can be a very healing experience for children and teens, as they are able to develop new relationships, try on new personalities, behaviors, and coping skills, as well as experience being included and a part of something positive.

References

Blalock, S., Lindo, N., & Ray, D. (2019). Individual and group child-centered play therapy: Impact on social-emotional competencies. *Journal of Counseling & Development*, 97, 238–249.

Bratton, S. C., Ceballos, P. L., & Ferebee, K. W. (2009). Integration of structured expressive activities within a humanistic group play therapy format for pre-adolescents. *The Journal for Specialists in Group Work*, 34(3), 251–275.

Chinekesh, A., Kamalian, M., Eltemasi, M., Chinekesh, S., & Alavi, M. (2013). The effect of group play therapy on social-emotional skills in pre-school children. *Global Journal of Health Science*, 6(2), 163–167.

Dillman Taylor, D., Meany-Walen, K. K., Nelson, K. M., & Gungor, A. (2019). Investigating group Adlerian play therapy for children with disruptive behaviors: A single-case research design. *International Journal of Play Therapy*, 28(3), 168–182.

Grant, R. J. & Turner-Bumberry, T. (2020). *Autplay therapy play and social skills groups*. Routledge.

Grant, R. J., Stone, J., & Mellenthin, C. (2020). *Play therapy theories and perspectives: A collection of thoughts in the field*. Routledge.

Hudspeth, E. F. & Matthews, K. (2016). Neuroscience and play therapy: The neurobiologically informed therapist. In O'Connor, K. J., Schaefer, C. E., & Braverman, L. D. (Eds.), *Handbook of play therapy* (2nd ed., pp. 583–597). Wiley.

Kottman, T. (2011). *Play therapy: Basics and beyond* (2nd ed.). American Counseling Association.

Kulic, K. R., Dagley, J. C., & Horne, A. (2001). Prevention groups with children and adolescents. *Journal for Specialists in Group Work*, 26, 211–218.

Landreth, G. L. (1991). Foreword. In Sweeney, D. S. & Homeyer, L. E. (Eds.), *The handbook of group play therapy. How to do it, how it works, whom it's best for* (pp. xi–xii). Jossey-Bass.

Landreth, G. L. (2016, September 16–17). *The art of the relationship in play therapy: Deeper issues.* UAPT Annual Conference, Salt Lake City, UT, United States.

Meany-Walen, K. K. & Kottman, T. (2019). Group Adlerian play therapy. *International Journal of Play Therapy*, 28(1), 1–12.

Meany-Walen, K. K., Bullis, Q., Kottman, T., & Dillman Taylor, D. (2015). Group Adlerian play therapy with children with off-task behavior. *Journal for Specialists in Group Work*, 40, 294–314.

Meany-Walen, K. K., Bratton, S. C., & Kottman, T. (2014). Effect of Adlerian play therapy on reducing student behaviors. *Journal of Counseling & Development*, 92, 47–56.

Mellenthin, C. (2020). Issues of non-compliance and aggression. In Grant, R. J., Stone, J., & Mellenthin, C. (Eds.), *Play therapy theories and perspectives: A collection of thoughts in the field* (pp. 110–119). Routledge.

Merrell, K. W. (2011). *Social emotional assets and resilience scales: Professional manual.* PAR.

Morshed, N., Babmiri, M., Zemestani, M., & Alipour, N. (2019). A comparative study on the effectiveness of individual and group play therapy on symptoms of oppositional defiant disorders among children. *Korean Journal of Family Medicine*, 40(6), 368–372.

Perryman, K. L., Moss, R., & Cochran, K. (2015). Child-centered expressive arts and play therapy: School groups for at-risk adolescent girls. *International Journal of Play Therapy*, 24(4), 205–220.

Perryman, K. L. (2016). Play therapy in schools. In O'Connor, K. J., Schaefer, C. E., & Braverman, L. D. (Eds.), *Handbook of play therapy* (2nd ed., pp. 485–503). Wiley.

Ray, D. C. (2011). *Advanced play therapy: Essential conditions, knowledge, and skills for child practice.* Routledge.

Rich, B. W., Molloy, P., Hart, B., Ginsberg, S., & Mulvey, T. (2007). Conducting a children's divorce group: One approach. *Journal of Child and Adolescent Psychiatric Nursing*, 20(3), 163–175.

Substance Abuse and Mental Health Services Administration. (2018, October). *National Mental Health Survey [M-MHSS]* 2018. U.S. Department of Health and Human Services. Retrieved from: www.samhsa.gov/data/sites/default/files/cbhsq-reports/NMHSS-2018.pdf.

Swank, J. M., Cheung, C., Prikhidko, A., & Su, Y. (2017). Nature-based child-centered group play therapy and behavioral concerns: A single case design. *International Journal of Play Therapy*, 26(1), 47–57.

Sweeney, D. S. & Homeyer, L. E. (1991). *The handbook of group play therapy. How to do it, how it works, whom it's best for.* Jossey-Bass.

Sweeney, D. S., Baggerly, J. N., & Ray, D. C. (2014). *Group play therapy: A dynamic approach.* Routledge.

Tuckman, B. W. (1965). Personality structure, group composition, and group functioning. *Sociometry*, 27(4), 469–487.

Webb, N. B. (2010). *Helping bereaved children* (3rd ed.). Guilford Press.

Woolf, A. (2011). Everyone playing in class: A group play provision for enhancing the emotional well-being of children in school. *British Journal of Special Education*, 38(4), 178–190.

Yalom, I. (1995). *The theory and practice of group psychotherapy* (4th ed.). Basic Books.

Part III
Special Populations

12 Group Play Therapy with Military Connected Children and Families

Anne L. Stewart and Lennis G. Echterling

In military families, every member "serves" and is impacted by the challenges, uncertainties, and risks that are part of the parent's military service. There are currently more than 1.2 million children with a parent serving in the military in the United States (The School Superintendents Association [AAAS], 2019). Studies have documented psychological health challenges for military-connected parents and children suggesting that families would benefit from interventions that promote attachment and resilience across the military community (Skomorovsky, 2019). In this chapter, we provide an overview of the unique circumstances of military families, describe the healing dynamics that a resilience-informed multi-family group format can offer through the lens of attachment theory, and present creative, culturally-responsive, and relevant play-based activities for military-connected children and families.

Overview

Military-connected families encounter worries that are similar to those who pursue civilian careers; however, distinct aspects of a military lifestyle lend additional stressors. In addition, it is important to understand that military personnel and their families have differing experiences depending on their branch of service, their military rank, and whether they are on active duty, part of a reserve unit, or a member the National Guard. Concerns about the general safety of the service member, anticipated and unexpected separations from home, frequent relocations, new communities, as well as joyful and disruptive reunions can all be part of a military-connected family's lifestyle (Stevens et al., 2017).

Although some investigations report positive outcomes associated with parental military service, such as increased adaptive coping in teenaged members (Huebner et al., 2007), the mental health outcomes associated with military-connected families (particularly families experiencing multiple deployments) are predominantly negative and include anxiety, depression, acting out behaviors, and academic problems (Skomorovsky, 2019).

Parents' experiences of military culture and deployment, such as reliance on routine or emotional numbness and hypervigilance, can interfere

DOI: 10.4324/9781003094531-12

with realizing positive parenting experiences (Creech et al., 2014; Stevens et al., 2017). Studies have shown that although service members who have been deployed may not meet criteria for PTSD, they often have elevated trauma symptoms and their spouses experience negative emotions, including anxiety, sadness, and loneliness. Therefore, interventions, such as group play therapy, that attend not only to the child, but to the relationships and emotional health of military parents, are vital.

Working with military children and families in groups offers a number of significant advantages (Julian et al., 2018), however, using group dynamics to promote well-being has been a relatively recent strategy in the mental health field. Initially, practitioners turned to using groups because the sheer numbers of those in need made it impossible to work with each client individually. Now meta-analyses of group studies have provided overwhelming evidence that group interventions as efficacious as individual therapy (Paturel, 2012).

Military children and family members participating in a group intervention can experience feelings of belongingness and affiliation with others who share their concerns. In their encounters with other children and parents, they observe other effective coping strategies, practice crisis resolution skills, and receive useful feedback and, importantly, realize that they are not alone in their experiences (Julian et al., 2018; Lester et al., 2012).

Especially relevant for our work is that play is an excellent vehicle for promoting children's emotional development and affective regulation. Interactive play with a caring adult is a natural conduit for children to realize many physical, social, and neurologic development potentialities and it serves as a pathway for enhancing regulation and interpersonal connections disrupted by acute or chronic stress and loss (Perry et al., 2000). Offering developmentally attuned and playful group interventions with children and families can provide an abundance of healing opportunities in the form of engaging moment-to-moment interactions. Each family helps build group cohesion, composing a relational narrative – collectively promoting attachment and building resilience. The information in this chapter applies to both groups comprised of military-connected children and groups using a multi-family group intervention format.

Theory and Research

Attachment theory and resilience have direct relevance to helping play therapists understand the challenges that may place military families at risk for increased parenting difficulties. *And* they offer helpful frameworks to implement relevant interventions to address these challenges. Military parents endorse a high level of stress related to parenting and are especially concerned about navigating extended and typical family separations, reunions, and loss – i.e., how to maintain healthy connections and relationships – the precise territory of attachment theory. In addition, the majority of military family research has identified the negative outcomes of service on military members and their families, however, a growing literature base is focusing on protective factors and positive outcomes for families, namely, advocating for a resilience model to guide interventions.

Attachment Theory

Attachment theory provides an evidence-based framework to conceptualize parent-child relationships within the military family. The theory emphasizes the importance of interdependent relationships and refers to the affectional bond formed between child and caregiver. The emotional bond is established through developmentally congruent and emotionally gratifying everyday interactions and ultimately results in an internal working model of the self and others that guides future interpersonal interactions (Bowlby, 1988).

The power of attachment-based interventions is the focus on helping the parent meet the child's basic relationship needs in the context of play-based interactions. Attachment theory posits that parents serve as the child's *safe haven* in times of psychological distress and as a *secure base* from which to explore. Acting as a safe haven, the parent helps soothe, reassure, and reestablish emotional safety for their child – engaging in ways to help co-regulate and calm their distress. As a secure base, the parent supports the child's exploratory needs for learning about themselves, other people, and their world. Parents succeed by being sensitive to or "attuned" to the child's emotional world; engaging in reflective functioning, where they simultaneously resonate with one another; and by actively assisting the child to co-regulate their emotions and behavior during moment-to-moment interactions (Whelan & Stewart, 2015). The long-term outcome of these brief, but significant, interactions is that the child's brain builds a progressively complex structure of neural connections that result in successful rhythms of soothing, co-regulation of thoughts, emotion, and behavior, and capacities for self-control, and behavioral and social competence (Whelan & Stewart, 2015).

An overarching goal of an attachment-informed multi-family play therapy group activity is to create openings for attuned and responsive interactions between children and parents (and play therapist), so that the child's feelings will become more internally congruent. Offering attachment-informed play-based interventions in group settings offers family members opportunities to explore, express, and process their emotions. By providing a safe haven, inviting shared experiences, encouraging nonverbal expression, and engaging family members in playful encounters, play therapists can combine the benefits of both play and group dynamics to energize children and family members, normalize reactions, empower their adaptive coping skills, and promote family well-being. From this perspective, creating a safe and secure relationship and being engaged in play are inextricably intertwined.

Resilience

Resilience is the ability to "bounce back" after adverse conditions and catastrophic events. Researchers have applied the concept of resilience to individuals, families, organizations, environments, and communities (Houston, 2015). These studies have found that resilience is much more common than was once assumed (Echterling & Stewart, 2008). Even in troubled times, people often demonstrate great resilience by relying on their personal strengths, ingenuity, and resourcefulness (Maurovic et al., 2020). Research has consistently found that several factors promote resilience among children and families: social support, making meaning, emotional regulation, and creative coping (Masten & Reed, 2002).

Social Support

Creating bonds with other humans is not only necessary for psychological well-being, it is also a fundamental need of human existence. Social support improves physical and mental health, promotes recovery from illness, and is particularly crucial for military families who are going through periods of high stress (Lester et al., 2012). Moreover, lack of social support, such as chronic loneliness, is a major risk factor for premature death – higher even than smoking and obesity (Holt-Lunstad et al., 2015. The human species evolved in small tribes that promoted a profound sense of belongingness. Even in war, the social support among combatants enhances tribal connectivity and psychological resilience (Junger, 2016).

Making Meaning

Military-connected children use expressive arts and play to weave together wordless stories that give meaning to their worries and distress. In the midst of their turmoil, adults also may find it therapeutic to engage in drawing to begin giving form to their chaotic experience. Later, they may develop narratives that include themes of personal discoveries, life lessons learned, and a deeper sense of coherence and meaning. Those who are successful in creating positive meaning during this process of resolution eventually demonstrate greater resilience in their lives (Park, 2017).

Emotional Regulation

Military-connected children and families often struggle with intense emotional distress, such as anxiety and grief, that confronts them in troubled times. In addition to these negative emotions, the potential for resilience is also evident in the emerging positive feelings of gratitude, compassion, and hope (Conway et al., 2013). Acknowledging, recognizing, and expressing these feelings are essential in effectively regulating emotions and developing resilience.

Creative Coping

In the midst of their troubles, military families work to resolve their crises by taking action to address the challenging circumstances that confront them. They often demonstrate amazing resilience by turning to the physical, familial, emotional, financial, and community resources they have at hand. As a result, resilient families not only survive troubled times, they go on to thrive in their lives.

Military families, like individuals, are resilient and can quickly begin a process of resolution. Although the principles, processes, and goals of group-based play therapy are similar to those of traditional individual play therapy, groups present different dynamics, challenges, and opportunities for therapists. One of the most important values of a multi-family group setting is that it provides a forum where families in crisis can begin to co-construct a collective survival story. Members create a group narrative by assembling the bits and pieces of their personal impressions into a collage of shared meanings. Revealing a family's story, recognizing one's own family experiences in the accounts of others, building on one another's metaphors, elaborating on common themes, and contrasting perspectives can transform solitary family narratives into an evolving group survival story. Co-creating meaning is an ongoing process, not a single epiphany. By helping families to begin co-constructing this narrative, play therapists can enhance the group's sense of cohesion and help members to develop a common mission.

Attachment and Resilience-Informed Case Consultation and Interventions

Using attachment and resilience as guiding frameworks, play therapists can engage in case consultation and create interventions that are especially meaningful for military-connected children and families. Play therapists are encouraged to be intentional about understanding the characteristics of military culture, including the norms and beliefs of individual service members and their families. The unique culture of the military requires play therapists to be aware of their own values, biases, preconceived notions, and limitations through engagement in self-reflection and clinical supervision.

In addition to military cultural considerations, it is important for play therapists to address broader cultural factors and social identities, as well as historical and contemporary racial trauma, as they design and conduct therapeutic play interventions. According to the Children's Defense Fund, in 2018, children of color made up[1] nearly 50% of the total US child population and more than half the child population in 14 states and the District of Columbia (Children's Defense Fund, 2020). It is important that play therapists ensure that the group play therapy experience will be inclusive, responsive, and meaningful to family members across race, ethnicity, class, ability, age, culture, nationality, sexual orientation, SES, religious beliefs, social identities, and diverse perspectives by acknowledging and honoring the values and traditions of military families.

Treatment is focused on children and families as they navigate relationships, transitions, change, and resiliency, not about political affiliations. Consider family, parent, and child characteristics and overall number of participants you wish to involve when creating a group, for example you may wish to group families with children of similar ages.

Case Consultation

The authors partnered with families with deployed members in an innovative play-based group intervention that included caregivers and children coming to share dinner (potluck format) followed by separate youth and adult gatherings. The group was hosted by the family liaison officer at a regional armory and included families with children from newborn to 17-years-old. The youth group adopted a consistent ice breaker activity followed by a mix of structured and free play, depending upon the age range and needs of the children present. The adult group meeting implemented a support group format, where family members shared concerns and resources. Family and extended family members and facilitators "broke bread" together each meeting, engaging in lively conversation about a wide range of topics, resulting in the establishment of trusting and warm relationships. Informal and more formal consultation about a variety of issues across the life span resulted.

As attendees talked in small groups before dinner, Lisa, mother of twin toddlers, approached me (AS) concerned about an intervention gone awry. Following a suggestion from a website about strategies to ease deployment separation, her spouse had created a video to play for their 15-month-olds after he departed. She shared that this was their first deployment and they just did not know how to tell the children about his leaving. They determined that having him deliver the news that he was away by video would be perfect – it would provide the information and they could see daddy! Unfortunately, the toddlers were now upset and confused, she reported, looking for daddy in the TV set. An empathic consultation with information about how hard it was to be separated and some concise information about typical child development, viz., children's ability to realize screen images represent their equivalents in the real world emerges around 18 months of age, helped Lisa better understand her own upset as well as that of her twins. Subsequently, the therapist was able to easily facilitate a connection to another family with preschool children resulting in respite care and reassurance for both worried caregivers.

Guided by dimensions of attachment (address *safe haven* and *secure base* needs) and resilience (providing *social support*, helping to *make meaning*, experiencing a *range of emotions*, and adaptively *coping*), we found we were able to offer relevant and meaningful support for family members – all in the context of a caring relationship formed over dinner.

Interventions

The integration of play therapy strategies and techniques in a group format targets the therapeutic powers of play to help prevent or resolve the psycho-social difficulties associated with military service and support continued growth and development. Taking time to discuss the experiential activities is optional and may be helpful with older children and teens. Almost all the activities described below may be adapted for use in a telehealth platform and would require sending lists or kits of the necessary materials.

Rituals and Routines

Children and families form dynamic systems of interdependence. Play therapists can use routines and rituals to connect family members, affirm a collective cultural identity, and celebrate the journey on which they have all embarked. Therapists ask families to share the rituals and routines that offer structure, meaning and connectivity in their family experience. These include day-to-day routines and those associated with holidays or special celebrations. Thus, it is especially important to create "hello" and "good-bye" rituals for the group.

Collaborating with military families to create session agendas can create a sense of ownership by addressing their concerns and needs. The agenda for each meeting should be followed consistently, but not rigidly. The use of an agenda permits families sufficient predictability to reduce their anxiety, to take risks in participating, to explore promising strategies for resilience and is consistent with the importance of routines in the military culture.

Mirror, Mirror

A playful and direct way to express attunement is through imitating the child's actions. The therapist invites parents to serve as a mirror for their child and follow their child's actions. On the count of three, the "mirroring" begins! A fun variation of this activity is for the parent to use the palm of their hand as a "hand mirror". The parent and child face each other and the parent attempts to keep the mirror in front of the child's face as the child moves. Each person takes turns being the leader and follower.

Warm Fuzzies

This activity provides family members with an opportunity to offer and receive positive feedback. Each group member has a small piece of fuzzy fabric and is invited to give a "warm fuzzy", in other words, share a compliment or positive comment, to a family member. The message is personal and highlights a quality that the giver especially appreciates. Keeping that warm fuzzy, the family member then offers another warm fuzzy to another person, along with a compliment. This process continues until everyone has had a turn in giving and receiving a warm fuzzy. If desired, the therapist may process this experience by asking, "What was it like for you to give, receive, and hear the messages that people shared here?" or "What discoveries did you make about yourself?" The therapist can use this part of the activity to respond empathically to family members' contributions, noting common themes that emerge, and exploring how they may apply this to their family's lives.

Create a Me Tree[2]

Group members are asked to consider what type of tree they would like to be. They create the tree and identify at least three positive qualities and place them on the roots by drawing words or symbols or using images and words from magazines. Next, family members identify three or more achievements and place them on the branches. Lastly, they place symbols or names of the people who helped them along on the trunk of the tree. An alternative is to use the roots to depict their family history; the ground to show where they live now and the activities they engage in during the day, and the trunk to illustrate skills and talents they possess. Branches show the hopes, dreams, and wishes for the family's future; the leaves represent people that are or have been important to them; and fruits can note the gifts they have been given (acts of kindness, care, love).

Like a Rock

Family members go on a walk and select rocks with characteristics that remind them of a pain, loss, trauma, or hurt they are experiencing and have endured. They are invited to decorate the rock with words or symbols that recall the personal strengths and/or people that help them survive and thrive. Members create a title on a card beside the rock and the group completes a "gallery walk" to view all the creations. A variation is to put a word of hope on the stone.

Mixed Media Messages

Have the child or family create a picture of a TV/computer/phone and fill in the words, messages, and/or pictures that they are seeing or hearing in the media related to racially traumatic events or their ethno-racial identity. Use the picture to start a discussion about how what is presented in the media can send confusing and upsetting messages about the family's ethno-racial identity. The play therapist can help the group members support each other as they identify and process the range of emotions and conflicting feelings. Create a new screen image and fill it with symbols and words promoting the positive customs and traditions of their own ethnic group and share the messages.

Holding Hands and Letting Go

The purpose of this exercise is to explore what family members want to hold on to/remember/keep and what they want to let go of/keep out of their lives. This could be used as a reflection or culminating activity for the group. Each family member requires paper and pencil and crayons or markers (or magazines and scissors to cut out words and images). Family members trace their own hands on a piece of paper. Inside one hand, they place the things they want to keep in their life, in words, symbols, or pictures. In the drawing of the other hand, they put things they are interested in letting go of or keeping out of their lives. An alternate version is to draw a heart on the page and put inside the heart people/ things/or lessons learned that they want to keep inside their heart, and on the outside, they put things they do not want to hold in their heart.

The therapist may invite the group to process the experience with the following prompts. How difficult or easy was it to choose the items? How strong is the boundary between what you want and don't want in your life? Which things are the hardest to let go of? Which will be the hardest to keep in? What experiences or people have brought these things into your life? What steps do you need to take to move forward toward having what you've represented?

Human Rock, Paper, Scissors

This is a full body expression of the traditional game of rock, paper, scissors played by a pair of people showing their fists in one of these forms. In the full body pose game, a rock is shown by bending down and hugging your knees to curl into a ball, paper is shown by standing with your arms straight up above your head and your feet shoulder-width apart, while the scissors pose is standing with legs shoulder-width apart and both arms up and hands behind the head to look like a pair of scissors. For each round, each family constitutes a team and will do the poses (everyone in the family will need to do the same pose). Families will have three minutes to strategize. Once the families have their poses ready, the play therapist will count down "three...two...one...GO". On "GO" each family team will strike one of the three poses. Best out of three or five rounds is a good number for a medium sized group.

Duck, Duck, Goose, Hug

One of the most elating and stimulating activities from childhood is being chased, eclipsed only by the thrill of being caught. *Duck, Duck, Goose, Hug* is a variation of the traditional chase game of *Duck, Duck, Goose* in which a person who is sitting in a circle is tapped from behind and then chases and tries to catch the person who tapped them. Instead, in this version the person is tapped and then runs around the group in the opposite direction so the two meet and then can hug.

Create a Safe Place

Being in nature can help children, teens, and family members with addressing complex trauma symptoms. Group members are asked to think of a time and outdoor space where they felt safe and secure. They are invited to recall their surroundings, the season, the scents, lighting, and temperature and then to think about what they saw around and the feelings that were evoked. After the families have their memory gathered, they collect items from nature that help recreate the feeling from that place and build a new safe place. Lastly, they may take a photo of their creation (or something that creates the secure, calm feeling) to keep with them.

An Imaginary Goodbye Gift

Eventually all military families contend with change and transition, which is often accompanied by various types of loss – the loss of their deployed parent, and losses such as loss of routine, loss of a sense of safety, and loss of special time with their parent (Hall, 2008). Thus, the activity to recognize the loss of the group play therapy time together is an essential consideration.

The *Imaginary Goodbye Gift* gives group members an opportunity to say "Goodbye" personally to one another in the last session of a group. Invite the family group members to share an imaginary goodbye gift to each other by saying, "If I could give you one thing, it would be…". The gift giver may also share their reasons for choosing the present. The gift may reflect the recipient's personality, talents, interests, or contributions to the family or the group meetings. The giver offers a gift to another family member or another person in the circle. The activity continues until everyone has had the opportunity to share and receive an imaginary gift. Processing questions could include "What was it like for you to share your goodbye gifts to the others?" "What was it like to receive these gifts?" "What else would you like to say to one another as we come to the end of our group?"

Conclusion

Working with military children and families in groups offers a number of significant opportunities for promoting attachment and resilience. In a therapeutic space, they exchange ideas and personal stories, and experience first-hand the normality of their own reactions. As they share their stories in a group setting, children and families receive and provide social support, explore perspectives and make meaning, and experience a range of emotions in the context of caring relationships. Children and families can share their distress in troubled times, conspire to generate creative ways to cope, and have fun together. Playful groups are not only efficient in promoting positive parent-child relationships and child and family resilience, but they are also powerful therapeutic tools.

Notes

1 Children of color include all racial categories except white.
2 Adapted from Malchiodi, C. (2015).

References

Bowlby, J. (1988). *A secure base: Parent-child attachment and healthy human development*. Basic Books.

Children's Defense Fund. (2020). *The state of America's children*. www.children sdefense.org/wp-content/uploads/2020/02/The-State-Of-Americas-Children-2020. pdf.

Conway, A. M., Tugade, M. M., Catalino, L. I., & Fredrickson, B. L. (2013). The broaden-and-build theory of positive emotions: Form, function, and mechanisms. In S. A. David, I. Boniwell, & A. Conley Ayers (Eds.), *The Oxford handbook of happiness* (pp. 17–34). Oxford University Press.

Creech, S., Hadley, W., & Borsari, B. (2014). The impact of military deployment and reintegration on children and parenting: A systematic review. *Professional Psychology Research and Practice*, 45(6), 452–464. doi:10.1037/a0035055.

Echterling, L. G. & Stewart, A. L. (2008). Resilience. In S. F. Davis & W. Buskist (Eds.), *Twenty-first century psychology: A reference handbook* (Vol. 2, pp. 192–201). Sage.

Hall, L. K. (2008). *Counseling military families*. Routledge.

Holt-Lunstad, J., Smith, T. B., Baker, M., Harris, T., & Stephenson, D. (2015). Loneliness and social relationships as risk factors for mortality: A meta-analytic review. *Perspectives on Psychological Science*, 10(2), 227–237. doi:10.1177/1745691614568352.

Houston, J. B. (2015). Bouncing forward: Assessing advances in community resilience assessment, intervention, and theory to guide future work. *American Behavioral Scientist*, 59(2), 175–180.

Huebner, A., Mancini, J., Wilcox, R., Grass, S., & Grass, G. (2007). Parental deployment and youth in military families: Exploring uncertainty and ambiguous loss. *Family Relations*, 56(2), 112–122. doi:10.1111/j.1741-3729.2007.00445.x.

Julian, M. M., Muzik, M., Kees, M., Valenstein, M., & Rosenblum, L. L. (2018). Strong Military Families intervention enhances parenting reflectivity and representations in families with young children. *Infant Mental Health Journal*, 39(1), 106–118.

Junger, S. (2016). *Tribe: On homecoming and belonging*. Hachette Book Group.

Lester, P., Saltzman, W. R., Woodward, K., Glover, D., Leskin, G. A., Bursch, B., Pynoos, R., & Beardslee, W. (2012). Evaluation of a family-centered prevention intervention for military children and families facing wartime deployments. *American Journal of Public Health*, 102, 48–54.

Malchiodi, C. (2015). *Creative interventions with traumatized children*. Guilford.

Masten, A. S. & Reed, M.-G. J. (2002). Resilience in development. In C. R. Snyder & S. J. Lopez (Eds.), *Handbook of positive psychology* (pp. 74–88). Oxford University Press.

Maurovic, I., Liebenberg, L., & Feric, M. (2020). A review of family resilience: Understanding the concept and operationalization challenges to inform research and practice. *Child Care in Practice*, 26(4), 337–357. doi:1080/13575279.2020.1792838.

Park, C. L. (2017). Distinctions to promote an integrated perspective on meaning: Global meaning and meaning-making processes. *Journal of Constructivist Psychology*, 30(1), 14–19. doi:10.1080?10720537.2015.1119083.

Paturel, A. (2012). Power in numbers: Research is pinpointing the factors that make group therapy successful. *APA Monitor*, 43(10), 48.

Perry, B. D., Hogan, L., & Marlin, S. (2000). Curiosity, pleasure and play: A neurodevelopmental perspective. *HAAEYC Advocate*. https://7079168e-705a-4dc7-be05-2218087aa989.filesusr.com/ugd/aa51c7_c8a5130ebf2e4cd184a6e5dc1d41feae.pdf.

Skomorovsky, A. (2019). Impact of military life on children from military families. *Journal of Military, Veteran and Family Health*, 5(2). https://jmvfh.utpjournals.press/doi/pdf/10.3138/jmvfh.2019.5.issue-s2.

Stevens, L., Hinesley, J., Stewart, A., Atwood, K., & Pickett, T. (2017). Relevance of attachment theory to parenting concerns among veterans with TBI and PTSD. *Current Treatment Options in Psychiatry*, 4(3), 241–253.

The School Superintendents Association. (AASA, 2019). *Fact sheet on the military child*. www.aasa.org/content.aspx?id=8998.

Whelan, W. F. & Stewart, A. L. (2015). Attachment-focused play therapy. In D. Crenshaw & A. L. Stewart (Eds.), *Play therapy: A comprehensive guide to theory and practice*. Guilford.

13 Early Play-Based Interventions for Children Following Disastrous Events

From Principles to Practice

Janine Shelby

Childhood exposure to adverse events is common. A preponderance of children encounter childhood adversity (Felitti et al., 1998), and the United Nations International Children's Emergency Fund (UNICEF, 2018) report more than 250 million children throughout the world live in areas impacted by violence. Over the past two decades, 7,547 natural disasters have affected millions of children globally (Ritchie & Roser, 2020), and approximately 14% of US youth are exposed to disasters (Substance Abuse and Mental Health Services Administration [SAMHSA, 2018]). To inform early psychological assistance programs, evidence-informed guidelines, such as the Psychological First Aid protocol (PFA; Brymer et al., 2006) or the "five essential elements" article (Hobfoll et al., 2007), provide broad principles for early intervention. However, child-focused interventionists often question specifically *how* to apply these tenets in developmentally sensitive ways. In this chapter, techniques are proposed for interventionists, from the perspective of an interventionist who has worked in more than a dozen countries. The strategies discussed here are intended to provide pragmatic, field-based intervention options for interventionists assisting young survivors following disasters, mass-scale violence, or other tragic events.

Overview of Play-Based Interventions in Early Intervention Guidelines

The *Psychological First Aid: Field Operations Guide* (PFA; Brymer et al., 2006) was developed to establish a safe, evidence-informed, post-disaster/terrorism intervention protocol. It was formed by an expert consensus panel based on findings from existing research related to early intervention objectives. The PFA manual is widely regarded as "the first, and most favored, early intervention approach" (Shultz & Forbes, 2014, p. 1). It contains eight core intervention "actions", which were described as follows:

- contact and engagement
- safety and comfort
- stabilization

DOI: 10.4324/9781003094531-13

- information gathering related to current needs and concerns
- practical assistance
- connection with social supports
- information on coping
- linkage with collaborative services.

Another prominent publication that described the five essential elements of immediate- and mid-term intervention (hereafter referred to as the five elements; Hobfoll et al., 2007), was highly influential in shaping the thoughts of policy makers, care providers, and scholars in many parts of the world. Its components have informed intervention/prevention efforts, including practitioners of the PFA protocol. The five elements were also distilled from the body of existing early intervention evidence. They were as follows:

- a sense of safety
- a sense of calm
- a sense of self- and community efficacy
- connectedness
- hopefulness.

Like the PFA manual, the five elements article emphasized adult interventions, but included notes pertaining to young survivors.

Play was explicitly recommended in the PFA and implied in the five elements article. However, the purpose, type, and role of play were variously described or left unclear. Other authors have articulated that expressive arts activities (e.g., singing, art, storytelling, and play) may aid young survivors because of their relaxing and stabilizing properties (Bisson & Cohen, 2006). In addition, several play-based, early intervention techniques designed to deliver CBT objectives with children have been proposed by the author and colleagues (Felix et al., 2006; Shelby, 2019). Group-based interventions were referenced in both the PFA manual and the five elements article.

Although the PFA manual and the five elements text provide valuable overarching principles for post-disaster intervention, these texts discussed broad tenets rather than detailed intervention techniques. This broad scope leaves gaps in technical guidance and makes research more difficult to conduct (Benedek & Fullerton, 2007; Dieltjens et al., 2014; Fox et al., 2012). Clearly, greater continuity between prevailing guidelines and developmentally sensitive, practical intervention techniques is needed.

Research

Though many psychotherapy interventions for trauma-exposed youth have strong research support, far less is known about the effectiveness of *early*

interventions with young survivors. In their review of post-disaster interventions for children, Pfefferbaum et al. (2014) found that a variety of
individual and group approaches (e.g., debriefings, exposure, humanistic
therapy, and eye movement desensitization) have been delivered, but the
most used techniques were cognitive behavioral in nature. These approaches tended to include psychoeducation, relaxation, coping, and social
support. Insufficient data, as well as the fact that several programs used
more than a single method of intervention, prevented Pfefferbaum and
colleagues from concluding that one approach was superior to any of the
others. A review produced by SAMHSA (2018) lists several prominent
post-disaster interventions, including the CBT strategies Pfefferbaum and
colleagues described, as well as social support, parental involvement, and
other CBT elements. Play-based interventions were not highlighted in the
review, but some play-based, culturally sensitive interventions have been
shown to be effective. For example, Tominaga (2014) found that interventions using traditional stories were helpful for young survivors of natural
disasters in both China and Japan. Shen (2002) reported positive outcomes
using child-centered play therapy in a control group study of Chinese
children following an earthquake. In terms of group-based intervention
research, Newman et al.'s (2014) meta-analysis revealed greater benefit for
recipients of individual rather than group interventions. Yet, practical
considerations (e.g., ability to reach more children, and more efficient use
of staff and economic resources), as well as the social support properties of
groups, have led many to recognize, as Pfefferbaum and Shaw (2013) did:
group work is "ideal" for offering psychoeducational interventions to
children and their caregivers.

Research for early post-disaster interventions continues to amass but is
not yet robust. In the meantime, there is general consensus that early
interventions with youth should emphasize immediate-term safety and
stabilization, while fostering resilience, coping skills, and social support.

Play-Based Group Early Interventions

In the remainder of this chapter, group, play-based strategies will be presented. These interventions can be implemented in formal, or naturally
occurring, group settings following disastrous events. Based on the prevailing best practice standards (i.e., the PFA manual of Brymer et al.,
[2006] and Hobfoll and colleagues' [2007] five elements article), several
means by which child-focused interventionists can translate early intervention principles into practice will be proposed. Table 13.1, Play-Based
Techniques for the PFA manual and Five Essential Elements, lists the
intervention strategies described in this chapter and how they correspond
to both of these practice guides. Some interventions described in this text
can be used to address more than one core action or essential principle.
These intervention techniques are presented as examples of ways in which

Table 13.1 Play-Based Techniques for the PFA manual and Five Essential Elements

Essential Elements	PFA Core Actions Related to the Essential Elements	Practical Application Techniques
Safety	**Safety and Comfort**	• Ambient Safety Messages • Rumor Drop-Box • The Knowing Tree
Calming	**Stabilization**	• Sensory Stations • Soothing Sessions • Targeting Caregiver Resources to Calm Children • Puppetry for Affect Regulation
Efficacy	**Information on Coping Connection with Social Supports**	*Self-Efficacy* • Coping Activities • Coping Box • Four Messages ***Community Efficacy*** • Role-Playing Community Relief Efforts
Connectedness	**Connection with Social Supports**	• Social Support Identification
Hope	**No Specific Core Actions**	• Hope Wall • Hope Bag • Guided Imagery

Essential Elements are described by Hobfoll et al., (2007); The PFA is written by Brymer et al., (2006)

the principles can be delivered in early intervention settings. They are not intended as a full intervention protocol or comprehensive list of corresponding techniques.

Safety

In the PFA manual, safety refers to immediate physical safety, as well as physical and emotional comfort. In the five elements text, the principle of safety refers to physical and psychological sense of safety, as well as objective safety and subjective sense of safety. This element encompasses young survivors' – often disrupted – belief in their caregivers' ability to protect them from adversity. In the five elements article, survivors' access to accurate information is highlighted as a potential means of decreasing exaggerated or inaccurate perceptions of threat.

Children's sense of safety is enhanced when they receive clear, age-appropriate information about the disastrous event and deaths/injuries. In an earlier publication (Shelby, 2019), a detailed protocol was presented to assist interventionists and caregivers as they inform youth of tragic events. There, the use of four "Rs": rarity (i.e., describe, if true, the relatively unusual nature of the event), reveal (i.e., provide a brief, developmentally appropriate description of what occurred), reassurance (i.e., emphasize current safety or relative safety, and adults' intent to provide protection and/or comfort), and the reason (i.e., using developmentally sensitive language, briefly explain why the event occurred).

To enhance survivors' sense of psychological safety and comfort in early intervention settings, *voiceless interventions* are often useful. Voiceless interventions involve highly visible or readily accessible activities and materials designed to promote sense of safety, calm, adaptive coping, and hopefulness, without the explicit aid of interventionists. These interventions may be particularly helpful in the immediate aftermath of tragic events, when survivors often congregate in naturally occurring groups. These interventions are also useful when survivors feel uncomfortable being directly approached by interventionists, or if cultural prohibitions hinder verbalization of negative experiences or emotions. Several voiceless interventions are presented here, as well as in additional sections of this chapter.

Ambient Safety Messages

Signage or announcements about the safety measures that are underway or completed in the intervention setting are simple ways to provide safety-related messages and reassurance. Information should be accurate, realistic, and developmentally appropriate.

Rumor Dropbox

A centrally located drop-box provides an opportunity for children or their families to anonymously ask safety – or mental health – related questions. After questions are reviewed by interventionists, responses can be provided via signage, announcements, texts, or routinely scheduled question-and-answer meeting times. This is often an effective way to discover and address rumors, myths, misunderstandings, and common questions that survivors may have difficulty or feel uncomfortable communicating directly to interventionists.

Knowing Tree

In this psychoeducational intervention, a drawing or picture of a tree is placed atop and attached to a blank sheet of paper the same size. The foreground page with the picture of the tree contains "window" squares at various points in the tree branches. Each window is cut on three of its four sides, such that it opens while attached to the fourth side of the square. On the forward-facing side of each window, a question or statement is written to reflect a concern or question children often have following disastrous events. Responses to these questions are written (i.e., prior to the intervention activity) on the sheet of paper in the background, behind the window, so that when the window is opened, the answer is revealed. Tying a piece of thread to each window not only makes it easier to pull open, but also generates additional enticement for children to explore the knowing tree's psychoeducational content. Windows might contain questions such as "*Will I always feel this scared?*"; "*Is it my fault?*"; or "*Is it normal to want to be near my parents all the time, now?*" Answers revealed when the windows are opened might include "*There are many things you can try to feel better*"; "*It is not your fault*"; and "*It is normal to feel the way you do.*" Illustrating the questions and answers improves the comprehension of young children or those with poor literacy. Questions and answers can be updated and discussed during group meetings.

Calming

In the PFA manual, calming and orienting emotionally overwhelmed survivors are referenced in the core action called stabilization, which is provided when needed. In the five elements, it is recognized that some degree of physiological reactivity is normal or adaptive following disastrous events. Prolonged or excessive physiological distress, however, may lead to impairment in functioning and is the target of intervention.

Sensory Stations

This technique, another voiceless intervention, involves the interventionist constructing several stations (e.g., tabletops, room corners, or other designated spaces), where different types of sensory materials are available for survivors. Stations should involve soothing tactile experiences (e.g., sand, cotton balls, buckets of tepid water, or stress balls), visually soothing images (e.g., pictures of serene settings, or amusing photographs), items with soothing olfactory qualities (e.g., flowers, essences, spices, or flavors reminiscent of positive experiences), and pleasant auditory stimuli (e.g., fountains or subtle chimes). The interventionists may structure the activity by asking survivors to sequentially rotate to other stations every couple of minutes until all stations have been visited. Alternatively, stations may be available for participants to use in an unstructured manner, wherein survivors can explore the sensory experiences at their own pace.

Soothing Sessions

Interventions that provide opportunities for developmentally salient soothing experiences are critically important to young children, whose physiological arousal level may be amplified during the initial post-disaster period. For youth whose caregivers are available, frequently scheduled soothing sessions can be helpful in restoring a sense of calm. For example, a child's favorite soothing experiences (e.g., being rocked, sung to, having a story read, or swaddled) can be provided during a specially designated time each day or several times each day, if necessary. Caregivers often benefit as much as their children do from this calming, grounding experience. When caregivers are not available, interventionists can assist and accompany children as they select and wrap themselves in blankets, hold stuffed animals, sit quietly in large, decorated boxes, or other comfortable designated spaces with an ambience of subdued lighting, soft music, or other comforting conditions. In disaster relief settings, this intervention can be routinely scheduled through-out the day (e.g., the first five minutes of every hour), which promotes a serene environment for both children and adults in the intervention setting.

Targeting Caregiver Resources for Calming Children

In the PFA manual and the five elements text, caregivers are encouraged to provide comfort and reassurance to their children, but not all caregivers have the psychological resources or pre-existing parenting skills to ade-quately meet their children's heightened needs during the immediate aftermath of tragic events. In these cases, it may be more practical to identify caregiver strategies with a high-likelihood of use and potential for high-impact with children (i.e., effective comforting strategies already included in caregivers' repertoires). Interventionists can help parents eval-uate the strategies they are most likely to provide and determine those most likely to yield maximal benefit to the children. For example, a care-giver who cannot yet tolerate hearing a child's tearful discussion of fears related to the tragic event would be encouraged to temporarily identify a reassuring response strategy that is within the caregiver's capacity to pro-vide. These strategies include, but are not limited to the following:

- verbal reassurance (e.g., "I am with you now and will do everything I can to keep you safe")
- physical affection or close physical proximity
- provision of comforting materials (e.g., a comforting blanket or toy)
- privileges (e.g., temporarily sleeping near caregivers, or spending extra time with people who comfort the child)
- verbalization of a hope-based trajectory (e.g., "We will get through this and find a way to feel better in the future")
- adherence to daily routines
- child-led play with caregiver.

After caregivers begin to provide two or three targeted reassurance meth-ods to their children, youth can reinforce their caregivers' behaviors by holding a parent-appreciation ceremony, wherein the children present drawings or certificates of gratitude to their caregivers for their assistance and support. Children may complete the parent-appreciation activities individually or as a group. Caregivers may learn or identify reassurance methods on an individual or group basis. A group appreciation ceremony hosted by children for their caregivers is suggested to enhance social support and help restore children's perceptions of adult efficacy. When possible, caregivers' repertoires of reassurance strategies can be expanded across time.

Puppetry for Affect Regulation

Puppetry can be an effective tool to help children regulate their emotions and tolerate distress. Using puppets to perform for a group of children, interventionists can portray a story about characters who seek advice about their posttraumatic reactions. Other puppets are introduced into the narrative, and they sequentially explain how to use various affect regulation skills (e.g., positive imagery, relaxation techniques, social support, and helpful cognitions/behaviors). When the circumstances are conducive to an interactive puppet show, puppets can encourage children to practice the skills after the main character learns each technique. Children can also teach their own caregivers about their new skills, or pretend to teach new puppet-characters, as they are introduced into the story narrative.

Self- and Community Efficacy

Efficacy is divided into two subcomponents, self and community. In the PFA manual, the core action, information on coping, resembles the self-efficacy piece of the five elements text, whereas the PFA core action, connection with social supports, is most closely aligned with the five elements' description of community efficacy. In the five elements article, both self- and community efficacy enhancement are described broadly. Efficacy includes a sense of control over one's own outcomes (e.g., use of adaptive coping and emotional regulation skills, managing trauma-related triggers, and adversity-related problem-solving), as well as the belief in the efficacy of others (e.g., caregivers) and efficacious social or community responses.

Strategies to Promote Sense of Self-Efficacy

Coping Activities

From a selection of sticky notes or index cards with pictures and/or labels identifying typically adaptive coping strategies, young survivors select methods they believe would be helpful. After selecting a strategy/behavior, young survivors can practice the technique. Caregivers may then be invited to participate as youth explain how they intend to use their selected strategies. Multiple strategies can be compiled in individualized coping menus, which youth keep for future use. In group settings, children can select desired strategies in an engaging way by retrieving items that depict various coping skills from unexpected places (e.g., trees, various locations in the disaster relief setting, or on a spinning office chair). As an alternate activity, youth can be asked to pass cards that depict coping strategies around a circle of peers. Each child must select a card perceived as helpful to the child, while avoiding cards with unhelpful strategies, before the time lapses (i.e., 5 seconds per child, such that a group of 10 youth would have 50 seconds to pass the cards around the circle). As another option, paper clips are fastened to pieces of paper cut into the shape of fish. Coping strategies are drawn or written on one side. Children pretend to fish by attaching magnetized poles to these "fish". They then discuss the coping strategy on the fish and whether or not it would be helpful to them.

Coping Box

Coping boxes can be created from a wide array of materials (e.g., a simple cardboard box or an elaborately decorated wooden treasure chest) to demonstrate a coping chest or tool kit. When opened, the coping boxes reveal a variety of coping and sensory-based items, such as kinetic sand, squishy rubber balls, cotton balls, play dough, items with fragrant smells, bubbles, pictures, calming messages written to oneself, encouraging messages from loved ones, and other content likely to assist with coping abilities and self-soothing. As access to materials permits, children can design and fill their own coping boxes or bags, which they keep for future use.

Four Messages

Joyner (1991) proposed that youth identify four helpful messages to themselves and imagine that the coping messages are playing repeatedly, as if they are looping on a recording device. A more modern version of this idea involves recording four short video or audio messages to oneself, which can either be used individually or shared between members of a family or group (with appropriate parental consent). When these video and audio clips are stored on adolescents' personal electronic devices, they can be replayed, as needed.

Strategies to Promote A Sense of Community Efficacy

Role-Playing Community Relief Efforts

Pictures of adults with a role in disaster-relief efforts or community safety can be posted in the intervention setting as a reminder of recovery efforts. These adults can also be invited to speak to groups of children to describe their roles in relief efforts and respond to questions. Costumes and coloring books that depict community workers provide opportunities for young children to draw or play about intervention efforts and vicariously experience rebuilding endeavors. In group activities, children can engage in pretend play based on the roles of rebuilders, first responders, or others involved in community relief efforts.

Connectedness

In the PFA manual, the core action called connection with social supports focuses on enhancing contact with sources of social support. In the five elements article, connectedness includes dyadic, familial, peer, and community social support activities, as well as ways in which trauma processing and adaptive skills can be enhanced vis-à-vis social interrelatedness.

Social Support

Eight types of social support were identified in the five elements article (Hobfoll et al., 2007), as follows: (a) emotional closeness, (b) social connections, (c) feeling needed, (d) reassurance of self-worth, (e) reliable alliance, (f) advice, (g) physical assistance, and (h) material support. One engaging way to teach youth about these types of social support, also used in an intervention by Layne et al. (2001), is by offering young survivors the opportunity to identify individuals who may provide some – even if not all – of the social support types. For example, youth can write the names of potential sources of social support on color-coded objects that correspond to each type of support. Colored wooden beads or flat popsicle sticks allows children to write or draw specific individuals who are available or can be recruited to provide each type of social support (e.g., blue may refer to emotional closeness, red may indicate advice-giving, and so forth). The beads are then strung together to form necklaces, bracelets, or some other keepsake. Wooden popsicle sticks can be used to construct an object. Because more sticks or beads produce a more elaborate object, youth are often incentivized to identify many sources or potential sources of social support. Group settings allow youth to show their social support keepsakes to peers and can be particularly engaging. After the group activities, youth keep their projects, which serve as tangible reminders of available or recruitable social support sources.

Sense of Hope

Though not listed as a core action in the PFA manual, enhancing a sense of hope is indirectly addressed via other core actions (e.g., safety and comfort, stabilization, coping, and social support). According to the five elements text (Hobfoll et al., 2007), retaining a sense of hope is centrally important to post-disaster adjustment.

Hope Wall

In this voiceless activity, the label "reasons I will get through this" is affixed to a chalk board, wall, or other identified space. A written notice should invite both children and adults to participate by writing or drawing the people, pets, beliefs, personal skills, or experiences that provide a reason to persist, despite the hardships they face (e.g., "because my sister needs me"; "because my parent would want me to"; "to care for my pet"; or "because I know I can survive this"). Materials (e.g., writing implements, sticky notes) should be readily available for survivors to contribute their own statements to the wall. Participation is voluntary, but even those who do not participate are likely to benefit from exposure to the inspirational messages and art others have posted on the hope wall. In addition, the wall provides a natural entry point for conversations between survivors and interventionists.

Hope Bag

Inspired by a technique used in an intervention for suicidal adolescents (Asarnow et al., 2017), this technique is modified to prompt adolescents' use of positive, futuristic thoughts in post-disaster contexts. Using a small bag or box, youth are asked to select items that represent who they love, who needs them, something about which they are proud or enjoy, and something they look forward to in the future. The collection of items that fill the individualized hope bags may include small stones, feathers, seashells, fuzzy balls, wooden miniatures, stickers (e.g., of pets, favorite activities, sports, milestones, or travel experiences), and other items. Blank paper is available to add individualized components to the hope bag. The bag can be decorated and sealed with miniature clips or rubber bands, and re-opened when reminders are needed regarding the value and future possibilities of their lives. This activity can be delivered to individuals, families, or groups.

Guided Imagery

Guided imagery can be a practical way to engage large numbers of youth in settings where materials or resources are scant, but it can also be an effective means to generate hopeful images. It is particularly useful in settings with few resources and a large number of children. As one form of post-disaster imagery, children whose communities are extensively damaged can be asked to imagine a small, but powerful, light that is contained within each of them. Youth are asked to imagine that the light is initially small and shines only enough to see what is immediately in front of them. Then, the light grows sequentially larger and larger, until they can see their rebuilt or new homes. As the light grows yet stronger, youth are asked to envision their new or rebuilt homes, streets, schools, and neighborhoods. After youth look at the new world they can see in their minds, youth are reminded that the special light is theirs to keep and use any time they need to see beyond their current realities. Younger children may benefit from taking turns sharing the content of their imagery aloud or drawing/writing about what they imagined. When materials are available, youth might create a "tower of hope" in the intervention setting by stacking and gluing items (e.g., paper cups or boxes) with drawings or brief descriptions of their imagined futures.

Case Example

After a flood caused significant damage to a small community, survivors gathered at the gymnasium that will serve as their shelter until it is safe for them to return home. The disaster relief team had previously entered, and the interventionists began setting up stations for emotional and physical relief. As the survivors entered the building, the first thing they saw was the hope wall. Inspirational messages and drawings to promote efficacy, hope, and a shared sense of survival filled the space. As the families began to line up to register for shelter, interventionists invited the children to come and play with the sensory stations. Children raced past their caregivers to explore the intriguing sensory stations set up at various locations across the gymnasium. Caregivers' relief was evident, as they saw their children relax again, and enjoy themselves, as they stroked the kinesthetic sand in the tactile-objects station, watched sand pour through hourglasses in the visual station, and listened to relaxing music through headphones at the auditory station.

After the families had registered and settled their belongings under their cots, the lunch service began. As they waited to receive their meals, a psychoeducational puppet show was performed by the interventionists. Coping skills were taught and practiced by both puppets and the audience. After lunch, soothing chimes alerted shelter residents that it was time for a ten-minute "soothing session". Caregiver-child dyads were invited to participate, either from their cots or near the child-focused corner. Many childless adults across the shelter also took advantage of the soothing session for themselves.

When the soothing session ends, interventionists invited the children to remain in the child-focused corner to participate in coping-based, efficacy-based, and hope-based play activities. For the next hour, adolescents played a coping game in which they select and pass cards with coping skills before the timer sounds. They giggled, discussed their selected strategies, and were able to form a bond with the other teens. Throughout the day, younger children engaged in free play, visited various coping or psychoeducational activity stations set up throughout the shelter, and observed the safety messages posted on the shelter walls. Interventionists roamed from station to station, engaging in organic conversations that stemmed from the activities at each station. Some residents contributed items to the rumor box, and responses were provided during the evening dinner service. The residents were invited to one final soothing session that evening. Finally, as dusk began to settle, the interventionist ended the day with an imagery activity, in which youth choose an object or part of nature that connotes strength (e.g., a mountain or an old tree), and then imagine the identified object's strength being embodied within them.

Conclusion

Until additional research emerges, child-focused interventionists must rely on early intervention best practice guides, research extrapolated from related evidence, and the collective wisdom of experienced early interventionists. This chapter proposed practical ways to use play-based, group activities to deliver some of the principles put forth in the PFA manual and the five elements article. For the legions of dedicated clinicians, who tirelessly spring to action in response to disastrous events, it is hoped this chapter has highlighted what the children who inspired the interventions demonstrated: wellbeing is possible in spite of adversity.

References

Asarnow, J. R., Hughes, J. L., Babeva, K. N., & Sugar, C. A. (2017). Cognitive-behavioral family treatment for suicide attempt prevention: A randomized controlled trial. *Journal of the American Academy of Child and Adolescent Psychiatry*, 56(6), 506–514. doi:10.1016/j.jaac.2017.03.015.

Benedek, D. M. & Fullerton, C. S. (2007). Translating five essential elements into programs and practice. *Psychiatry*, 70(4), 345–349. doi:10.1521/psyc.2007.70.4.345.

Bisson, J. I. & Cohen, J. A. (2006). Disseminating early interventions following trauma. *Journal of Traumatic Stress*, 19, 583–595. doi:10.1002/jts.20175.

Brymer, M., Jacobs, A., Layne, C., Pynoos, R., Ruzek, J., Steinberg, A., Vernberg, E, & Watson, P. (2006). *Psychological first aid: Field operations guide* (2nd ed.). National Child Traumatic Stress Network and National Center for PTSD. www.nctsn.org.

Dieltjens, T., Moonens, I., Van Praet, K., De Buck, E., & Vandekerckhove, P. (2014). A systematic literature search on psychological first aid: Lack of evidence to develop guidelines. *PLoS ONE*, 9(12), e114714.

Felitti, V. J., Anda, R. F., Nordenberg, D., Williamson, D. F., Spitz, A. M., Edwards, V., Koss, M. P., & Marks, J. S. (1998). Relationship of childhood abuse and household dysfunction to many of the leading causes of death in adults: The Adverse Childhood Experiences (ACES) study. *American Journal of Preventive Medicine*, 14(4), 245–258. doi:10.1016/S0749-3797(98)00017-8.

Felix, E., Bond, D., & Shelby, J. S. (2006). Coping with disaster: Psychosocial interventions for children. In C. Schaefer & H. Kaduson (Eds.), *Contemporary play therapy: Theory, research, and practice* (pp. 307–326). Guilford.

Fox, J. H., Burkle, F. M., Jr., Bass, J., Pia, F. A., Epstein, J. L., & Markenson, D. (2012). The effectiveness of psychological first aid as a disaster intervention tool:

Research analysis of peer-reviewed literature from 1990–2010. *Disaster Medicine and Public Health Preparedness*, 6, 247–252.

Hobfoll, S., Watson, P., Bell, C. C., Bryant, R. A., Brymer, M. J., Friedman, M. J., Friedman, M., Gersons, B. P. R., de Jong, J. V. M., Layne, C. M., Maguen, S., Neria, Y., Norwood, A. E., Pynoos, R. S., Reissman, D., Ruzek, J. I., Shalev, A. Y, Solomon, Z., Steinberg, A. M., & Ursano, R. J. (2007). Five essential elements of immediate and mid-term mass trauma intervention: Empirical evidence. *Psychiatry*, 70(4), 283–315.

Joyner, C. D. (1991). Individual, group, and family crisis counseling following a hurricane: Case of Heather, age 9. In N. B. Webb (Ed.), *Play therapy with children in crisis* (pp. 396–415). Guilford.

Layne, C. M., Pynoos, R. S., Saltzman, W. R., Arslanagic, B., Black, M., Savjak, N., et al. (2001). Trauma/grief-focused group psychotherapy: School-based postwar intervention with traumatized Bosnian adolescents. *Group Dynamics-Theory Research and Practice*, 5, 277–290.

Newman, E., Pfefferbaum, B., Kirlic, N., Tett, R., Nelson, S., & Liles, B. (2014). Meta-analytic review of psychological interventions for children survivors of natural and man-made disasters. *Current Psychiatry Reports*, 16(9). doi:10.1007/s11920-014-0462-z.

Pfefferbaum, B. & Shaw, J. A. (2013). Practice parameter on disaster preparedness. *Journal of the American Academy of Child and Adolescent Psychiatry*, 52(11), 1224–1238.

Pfefferbaum, B., Sweeton, J. L., Nitiéma, P., Noffsinger, M. A., Varma, V., Nelson, S. D., & Newman, E. (2014). Child disaster mental health interventions: Therapy components. *Prehospital and Disaster Medicine*, 29(5), 494–502. doi:10.1017/S1049023X14000910.

Ritchie, H. & Roser, M. (2020). *Natural catastrophes*. Retrieved Dec. 31, 2020 from https://ourworldindata.org/grapher/natural-disasters-by-type?tab=table&time=2003.

Shelby, J. S. (2019). Play interventions for young survivors of disaster, terrorism, and other tragic events. In H. G. Kaduson, D. Cangelosi, & C. E. Schaefer (Eds.), *Prescriptive play therapy: Tailoring interventions for specific childhood problems* (pp. 107–126). Guilford.

Shen, Y. (2002). Short-term group play therapy with Chinese earthquake victims: Effects on anxiety, depression and adjustment. *International Journal of Play Therapy*, 11(1), 43–63.

Shultz, J. M. & Forbes, D. (2014). Psychological First Aid: Rapid proliferation and the search for evidence. *Disaster Health*. 2013 Aug 2; 2(1), 3–12. doi:10.4161/dish.26006.

Substance Abuse and Mental Health Services Administration (SAMHSA; 2018). *Disaster technical assistance center supplemental research bulletin: Behavioral health conditions in children and youth exposed to natural disasters.* www.samhsa.gov/sites/default/files/srb-childrenyouth-8-22-18.pdf.

Tominaga, Y. (2014). [*Psychological support for children after disaster/incident: A systems configuration and the guide to practice.*] Sogensya. (Japanese).

United Nations International Children's Emergency Fund (UNICEF, 2018). Children in war and conflict. *UNICEF USA*. Retrieved Nov. 4, 2020 from www.unicefusa.org/mission/emergencies/conflict.

14 Play Therapy Groups with Children of Divorce

A Jungian Approach

Eric J. Green and Karen Herdzik

Understanding the unique psychological effects of divorce on children are critical for play therapists to practice competently with this demographic. Clinical interventions for children whose families are dissolved and altered following a divorce should be carefully selected to help mitigate children from adverse long-term effects. The role of play therapy and the integration of experiential techniques can be useful in treatment when working with children affected by divorce (Green et al., 2019; Judge & Bailey, 2017). Specifically, group play therapy is one potentially beneficial modality. It supports children of divorce by increasing access to care and provides a unique opportunity for children to interact with and relate to peers facing similar concerns. In group psychotherapy, children learn from one another, feel less alone in their struggles, help each other find new solutions to old problems through creative means, and develop confidence in their ability to relate with others (DeLucia-Waack, 2006; Yalom & Leszcz, 2005). Group psychotherapy programs for children of divorce effectively reduce distress symptoms and improve children's communication in relationships with their parents (Pedro-Carroll, 2005). This chapter will examine the practice of group play therapy with children affected by divorce from a Jungian perspective. The Jungian group intervention permits children the opportunity for an integrative, salubrious experience to express feelings and activate self-healing potential through symbolic means via sandplay, group artwork, and mandalas. It concludes with parents being integrated into the therapeutic process to improve communication with their children. The next section will include an overview of children affected by divorce and how group play therapy may support their post-divorce mental health adjustment.

Overview

Children affected by divorce may experience deleterious psychological effects that negatively impact their well-being. Parental conflict can damage or impede a child's ability to form secure attachments with caretakers. Unfortunately, divorce often comes with endless, uphill battles of child custody

DOI: 10.4324/9781003094531-14

between the parents. In the United States, the family court system does not help to decrease the intensity of the custody battle, often ending in hostility and rejection toward one parent by the ex-spouse. A loyalty conflict within the child can arise when parents separate or divorce, especially in a hostile manner. Choosing one parent can decrease the child's cognitive dissonance resulting from the loyalty conflict (Bernet, 2020). According to the Divorce-Stress-Adjustment Perspective (Rosenberg, 2011), the divorce or splitting of a couple is a process that leads to many stressful events for the broken couple and especially the children. The severity or intensity of these stressful events and emotional factors depend on several moderating, protective factors. Protective factors refer to the actual resources available, the perspective of what divorce means, and the family's demographic characteristics. An increase in the presence and accessibility of protective factors decreases the likelihood of the stressful event impacting the child negatively. In other words, the company and the strength of protective factors determine how the child experiences a stressful event. In contrast, an increase of stressors correlates with mediating factors of loss of contact with one parent, the decline in parental support, and conflict between the parents post-divorce. The child's proliferation of stress can have long-lasting psychological effects on the child and can influence their ability to form attachments and adjust (Amato, 2000).

Children with attachment disorders are found among families coping with the aftermath of divorce. Due to the intense conflict, many parents tend to turn away, reject, or ultimately ignore the child's emotional needs. By not meeting the child's needs, the parent-child relationship and the quality of parenting suffers greatly, which directly leads to more child socio-emotional problems (Davies & Woitach, 2008). In a study by Sandler et al. (2008), both parents' warmth was studied per the child's perspective and experiences of living with or interacting with either parent. From these reports, the researchers also measured the internal and external problems that each child held. The results of the study showed the astonishing benefit of warmth from both parents. When the warmth of both parents was high, internalizing problems were found to be lower in children.

In contrast when both parents' warmth was low, the internalizing problems increased significantly, as expected. However, the high warmth of one parent is not sufficient for the child's emotional needs. Because of the lack of warmth of one parent, the dual task of providing emotional support becomes solely the job of the parent willing to provide warmth for the child (Sandler et al., 2008). This puts even more stress on the parent-child relationship and affects the child's ability to form secure attachments (Davies & Woitach, 2008; Sandler et al., 2008).

Children with parents negatively impacted by divorce may feel displaced or a sense of loss because their role has changed from a child to a miniature adult (Green et al., 2019). Harmful parenting and growing up in an unstable home environment are the primary variables that initiate poor outcomes related to parent-child attachment problems. These children tend to view their world as dangerous, unpredictable, and unsafe. The effects of insecure or disorganized attachments on children because of abusive or compromised parenting can be deleterious, particularly in interpersonal relationships. Children are also at risk of affect dysregulation, including frequent oppositional and aggressive behavioral problems (i.e., relational aggression) (Chambers, 2017). Because of family disruption and stresses before, during, and after a high-conflict divorce, some children may feel responsible or emotionally and physically compelled to console their caretakers' unmet needs. If not intervened appropriately, mild and moderate cases of parent-child contact problems can morph from developmentally appropriate parent-child alignment into unhealthy severe parent-child alignment (Fidler & Ward, 2017; Green et al., 2019).

The use of play and experiential therapies in treating families with difficult contact problems from varying degrees (i.e., mild, moderate, and severe) offers an alternative to traditional talk therapy between practitioners and families (Green et al., 2019). Play therapy is distinguished from other forms of treatment because it permits the child to create a world that constitutes a place of belonging, including safety from feeling shamed, judged, or banished. More importantly, play therapy principles can foster a therapeutic alliance built upon a trusting, emotionally safe (i.e., non-threatening and non-judgmental) relationship between the child and the therapist (Green, 2014). The warmth and comfort of a trusting relationship can help 1) cultivate a therapeutic bond of empathy that empowers the child to practice self-compassion toward themselves and others, 2) establishes safety and stabilization, 3) creates a place for safe expression, 4) carefully challenge and correct any distorted or inaccurate thoughts, and 5) reunify and recover connections with former relationships (i.e., less favored parent and extended family members) (Green, 2014; Green & Myrick, 2014; Judge & Bailey, 2017).

Additionally, an essential component of integrating experiential therapies in treatment is to reduce overwhelming anxiety, feelings of extraordinary stress, defensiveness, and alienation toward the less favored parent. Thus, the therapeutic reasoning for utilizing an integrative approach in divorcing/divorced familial dynamics can help children make meaningful connections with internal and external experiences, strengthen secure attachment bonds, and promote new relational patterns that foster safe disclosure (Green & Myrick, 2014; Judge & Bailey, 2017). van der Kolk (2014) described this interaction as *the visceral experience of reciprocity* for parents (and children) to learn and reunify their relationship to become emotionally and physically attuned. A significant component of experiential therapies and the role of play highlights the neurobiological benefits in family treatment. Mental health clinicians can incorporate developmentally age-appropriate approaches (i.e., Jungian group play therapy) into empirically supported psychotherapy approaches with children and families in divorce. Integrating play and experiential therapies can also help youth affected by divorce become more mindful and therefore *grounded* or *embodied*, increase creative self-expression, and develop improved communication with one or both parents (Green, 2014; van der Kolk, 2014).

Theory on Group Work with Children Affected by Divorce

Group psychotherapy programs to support children of divorce increase care access and provide a unique opportunity for children to interact with and relate to others facing similar concerns. In group psychotherapy, children learn from one another, feel less alone in their struggles, help each other, and develop confidence in their ability to relate with others (DeLucia-Waack, 2006; Yalom & Leszcz, 2005). Group psychotherapy programs for children of divorce effectively reduce distress symptoms and improve children's relationships with others (Pedro-Carroll, 2005). There is no consensus supporting a particular model of group psychotherapy for children of divorce as being more effective than others (Poli et al., 2017; Pollet, 2009). While there are different types of group play therapies, this chapter will focus on a Jungian perspective, psychodynamic treatment. Analytically-oriented treatments focus on expressing and understanding feelings and emotions (as opposed to concentrating on thoughts); exploring present-moment processes in session as a means of heightened self-awareness, providing a positive experience within the therapeutic relationship, and use of fantasy to evoke greater understanding and a creative approach to problem-solving. Analytic therapy typically prioritizes the child's affective experience (as opposed to external expectations or observations). Given the grief, stress, and relational strain children of divorce experience, analytically informed therapy can provide the needed opportunity to express and understand feelings, experience validation in a supportive relationship, and draw on creativity and imagination to navigate difficult times. Psychodynamic therapy is as generally useful as, and in some cases, more effective than cognitive-behavioral and other treatments (Shedler, 2010). While other analytically informed treatments can help children of divorce, Jungian play therapy in group formats has several features that make it particularly useful for children coping with typical or low-conflict divorce. Before we address these features, we will summarize Jungian play therapy's unique aspects below as a creative means of therapeutic engagement with children ages 5–13.

Jungian Play Therapy

Children learn about communication, emotional regulation, building relationships, moral judgment, how to deal with stress, develop their sense of Self, and prepare for life (Bludon et al., 2011). From an analytic perspective, play is essential to creativity in discovering and developing the whole Self. Jungian play psychotherapy is derived from the Greek word "psyche", which means "soul", and "therapei", which means "care of", so psychotherapy translated literally is "care for the soul". Green (2014) stated Jungian play therapy is the care of the entire Self of the client during which the therapist maintains a reverent stance for the innate wisdom in the Self of the client. Therapists create a *temenos* or sacred space where it is safe for the child to express and explore aspects of the unconscious through play and various other forms of self-expression (i.e., drawing, sandtray, storytelling, puppet theater, etc.). This temenos is physical, temporal, and relational. As the child plays, the therapist emotionally contains the child's experience by engaging in the child's experience, letting the child lead, and providing safety and reassurance when needed. Through therapy, the child accesses symbols and archetypes and builds the connection between their Ego and their Self and the collective unconscious. In doing so, the child accesses their innate ability to self-heal or their self-healing archetype. As the child expresses aspects of their Self, the therapist may amplify a symbol by eliciting the child to dialogue and play with the symbol.

Intervention: Jungian Group Play Therapy with Children Affected by Divorce

Jungian group play therapy with children affected by divorce is an integrative intervention, combining the symbolic and creative play-based modalities of coloring mandalas, sandplay, drawings, group artwork, and creating fairytales, with didactic, evidence-informed worksheets from a cognitive-behavioral perspective, specific to helping children cope with divorce. The materials needed are 1) the workbook, "Getting through My Parent's Divorce", by Baker and Andre (2018); 2) various art materials, including colored pencils/markers/crayons, glue, scissors, construction paper, long sheets of poster size white paper, glitter, etc., 3) miniature sand trays with sand in each sand tray, and assorted sand miniatures, and 4) age-appropriate, pre-drawn mandalas for coloring. Next, the selection process should include children close in age (within three years), groups no larger than 3–4 children, and children whose parents engaged in a low-conflict divorce. Medium to high-conflict divorces, which sometimes include parental alienation, lengthy and highly combative court proceedings, and/or complete disruption of the relationship between the child and one of the parents, are not appropriate for this modality. The duration of this intervention ideally should occur once per week for 16 weeks.

The process is divided into three archetypal codifications. Each one is sequential and approximately 4–6 weeks in length: *Fire, Water, Wind, and Earth*. More detailed information about how each of the components is practically implemented is in Table 14.1. Each 45-minute session begins with an entrance into the sacred space: a couple of minutes of yoga poses, relaxation through deep breathing, and check-ins. For the next 20 minutes, the children are instructed to produce either an individual sand picture, color a mandala, or complete a group drawing. The last 20 minutes is the

Table 14.1 Outline of Jungian Group Play with Children Affected by Divorce

Fire	Water	Wind	Earth
Weeks: 1–4	Weeks: 5–8	Weeks: 9–12	Weeks: 13–16
Creative: Group Art	Creative: Sandplay	Creative: Mandalas	Creative: Incorporating Parents into Play
Workbook: Activities 1–7	Workbook: Activities 8–13	Workbook: Activities 14–24	Workbook: Activities 25–33
Goal: Relationship Building/ Psychoeducation on Divorce/Coping Skills	Goal: Encouraging Yourself/Living Your Values/ Acting with Courage	Goal: Integrating Coping Skills for Optimal Post-Divorce Adjustment	Goal: Child-Parent Communication and Cohesion
Theme: Normalizing Feelings from Divorce	Theme: Social Reinforce- ment & Increas- ing Protective Processes	Theme: Finding Relief from Stress	Theme: Incor- porating Parents into the Process

didactic part, which involves 1–2 activities from the Baker workbook (see Table 14.1). The final minutes are used to transition the children back into the external world by playing music, usually accompanied by dance. The next section describes each of the creative modalities integrated into the Jungian group play therapy process with children affected by divorce.

Individual Sandplay

The children's individual sandplay work should be administered by a play therapist with training in sandplay from the *Sandplay Therapists of America* and have completed their supervised process in sandplay with a credentialed sandplay therapist or a personal process with a Jungian analyst. This component involves children producing sand imagery over a period of time. Specifically, children are instructed to create their own sand picture any way they would like using the sand miniatures available (see Figure 14.1). The group is advised to remain silent while completing their pictures. After everyone is done, children are given a chance to comment on their own sand picture, briefly. There are no follow-up questions or interpretations provided by the play therapist or any group member. The focus of this expressive modality is for children to feel grounded and embodied within the session. Sandplay permits the child a safe and protected space to create a projection of their interior life. The play therapist honors this sand picture creation, and each group member walks around the sand picture and observes it or "honors it" in silence. Children can

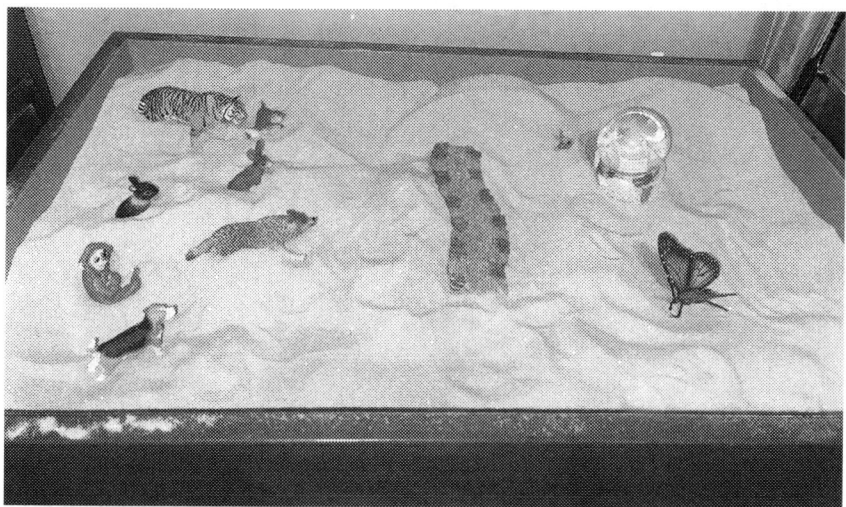

Figure 14.1 Sandplay Picture
Source: Image courtesy of Eric Green

comment on what they created if they choose. If they decide not to comment, the play therapist thanks the child for sharing their sand picture and moves on to the next child. The sand creations often depict the child's inner and outer realities as they matriculate through the divorce process. The kinesthetic action of manipulating sand can also be soothing and relaxing for a child. Sandplay used with children affected by divorce increases communication between child and parent; assists the child in developing solutions creatively to reoccurring problems related to the new family structure that may otherwise be too difficult to remediate through traditional talk therapy alone, and decreases anxiety and insecurity the child may be feeling in the post-divorce adjustment phase (Connolly & Green, 2009). The group learning component involved in incorporating sandplay is that children begin to identify others like them going through similar experiences. The existential feelings of loneliness are therefore diminished, and coping skills are increased.

Coloring Mandalas

Coloring mandalas is a relaxation technique used in Jungian group play therapy that is developmentally appropriate for children of all ages. Mandalas are circular shapes with designs inside them (see Figure 14.2). The play therapist presents the children with an assortment of mandalas and allows them to select the one they want and color it. Each mandala activity is given 15 minutes in total. After the children finish their mandalas, they are asked to tell the mandala's story or write it on the back of their coloring sheet. The play therapist does not ask intrusive questions after each child shares. This

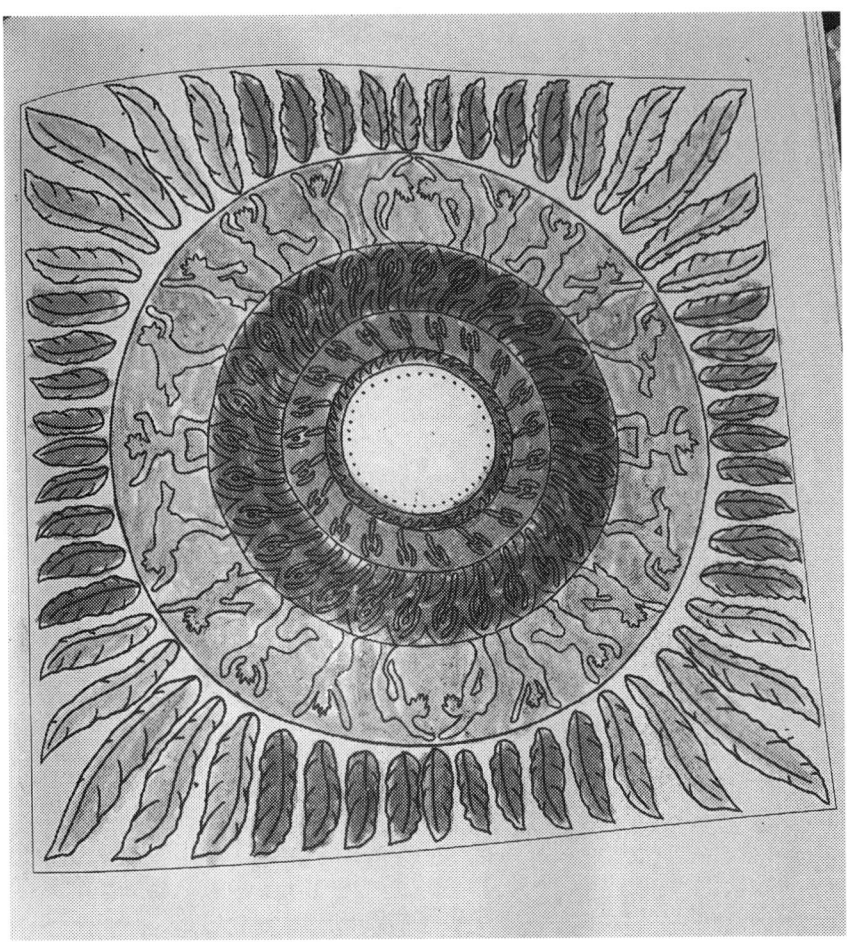

Figure 14.2 Mandala Drawn in Group Play Therapy
Source: Image courtesy of Eric Green

activity provides a grounding or embodied experience for each child by producing an original art creation, then sharing it with their peers in a psychologically safe space with no judgment. Each group member is advised not to
ask questions. Still, they are permitted to provide follow-up comments such
as, "Thank you for the effort you placed in your mandala", "I appreciated
you sharing your art with the group", or "I enjoyed the colors you used and
the story you told – it was creative. Thank you." Mandalas, like sandplay, are
done once per group session or every 2–3 sessions, depending on time considerations and the group dynamic. The play therapists keep all art until the
end of the group experience, then distribute the children's art to them if they
request it. The group learning from this activity is that children affected by

divorce learn coping skills through art and can share their creativity in a non-judgmental space, bringing about feelings of relaxation and acceptance.

Group Art

When a group art drawing is generated, the play therapists provide each individual member of the group 2–3 minutes to draw on a large piece of white paper, one at a time. The drawing's topic cannot be discussed beforehand; it is organic. Therefore, each child builds off the picture of the previous child. The activity can be a light-hearted activity that increases group cohesion. Another more structured group drawing is called "The 4 Elements". In this activity, each child's body is outlined on a large piece of paper. The four archetypal elements – Earth, Water, Wind, and Fire – are illustrated on the child's body outline or anywhere on the paper by the child. After each child completes the drawing, group sharing takes place. The play therapist discusses the importance of children reconnecting to nature, especially during the sometimes-unpleasant experiences correlated with a familial divorce. Therefore, an archetypal education is provided (see Appendix: Handout 1), giving children an opportunity to link the four archetypal elements with feelings they might be having regarding the divorce and their changing family dynamics. For example, each child is asked to describe *Wind* – a cooling event – a breeze; perhaps, they are asked to conceptualize when they feel soothed or what they can do to self-soothe. The four elements, or archetypal themes, are linked to internalized feelings and externalized experiences so that children develop an appre-ciation of the *symbolic attitude* or the awareness of linking their interior to the exterior through creative means, where healing occurs. This connection strengthens the child's ability to regulate affect, permitting children more opportunities to approach aberrant and difficult experiences stemming from divorce in a mindful, creative manner.

Parent Involvement

Parents who are simultaneously receiving their individual counseling or joint sessions to support co-parenting are invited to attend the group process during the last month. During each session, parents can observe, participate, and co-create play-based and creative designs with their children within the group format for the first 20 minutes. Parents are also involved with the didactic component-based element from the Baker workbook for the last 20 minutes, which provides information about how to best support their children in the post-divorce adjustment timeframe. This also gives parents an opportunity to be supervised in-vivo on parent-child communication by the play therapist.

Case Example

Two females, both ten years old, "Tenesha" and "Audrey", were screened and identified as appropriate to form a small play therapy group due to the similarities in their recent family dissolution surrounding their parents' low-conflict divorce. Tenesha was an only child whose parents divorced recently due to the father's infidelity. After her father had moved out of the family home, Tenesha began to exhibit depressive symptoms such as having trouble sleeping, feeling sad, and refusing to attend school at times. Tenesha's grades had also begun to suffer. Before the divorce, Tenesha and her father had enjoyed a secure attachment, with her dad often taking her to the park on weekends to play, as well as enjoying regular family movie nights, where they took turns choosing the film. Her father had recently moved out of state to be with the woman whom he had an affair with, and Tenesha now saw him infrequently.

Audrey's parents had also recently divorced due to financial troubles. Audrey previously experienced a secure attachment with both parents, but when she and her mother moved into a new home, she felt anger towards both parents. She would often be resistant to doing chores, which she previously enjoyed, like helping her mom clean the house during the week. She also got into a physical fight with a classmate at school one day over the classmate spilling Audrey's chocolate milk. These behaviors, along with her increasing aggression, were not present before the parental divorce.

During weeks 1–4, I (the first author of this chapter) worked with both girls to relationship-build and set an atmosphere of both safety and trust in the playroom. The girls quickly bonded by playing together. Specifically, we completed the "4 Elements" group art activity, and the girls saw how they were being impacted by the negative emotions surrounding their parent's divorce in similar ways. At one point, Tenesha commented, "I thought I was the only one that felt this way. Audrey feels sad sometimes, too." During weeks 5–12, we completed a play therapy or creative art activity, as outlined in Table 14.1. The children produced a series of individual sandplay pictures, as well as created mandalas. I also would divide each group play session into two, with the first half being the creative intervention and the second half being a correlated worksheet from the divorce workbook (Baker & Andre, 2018). The group engaged in discussions on coping skills to use for feelings of anxiety, stress, depression, and anger. Audrey found this part of our group work especially beneficial as her mother reported her aggression began to decrease at home toward both parents. The mandalas the girls created also provided insight into their processing not only conflictual feelings related to their family's dissolution but also themes of hope, optimism, and resilience surfaced.

During the final three or so weeks of the group, Audrey's mother and Tenesha's father participated in the sessions. The group worked on improving child-parent communication and cohesion by role-playing via puppet shows. The girls also requested they complete a sand picture and mandala while their parents watched. We continued incorporating the didactic pieces from the workbook, and both girls demonstrated positive outcomes as evidenced from a pre- and post-test and from parent reporting of their behaviors at home and school. Tenesha and her father had a breakthrough during treatment: he apologized to her for moving out of state and promised he would start calling and visiting more often. Audrey and her mother also began improving their attachment through the sandplay work as Audrey's mom, for the first time, was able to see the world from her child's creative sand expressions and no longer saw her as defiant and difficult, but needing more positive discipline, empathy, and attention. We ended the group at week 16, with both girls reporting feeling better within their relevant situations and relationships with their parents.

Conclusion

From an analytic perspective, which emphasizes parent-child relationships as foundational to the psychological well-being of the child, the grief and stress of parental divorce can threaten a child's sense of security in getting their needs met, their ability to develop realistic relational schema, and their ability to integrate and understand their own feelings (Gabbard, 2017). To assist children affected by divorce from a mental health standpoint, group play psychotherapy is one potentially beneficial modality employed by mental health clinicians to reduce distress symptoms and improve children's relationships with their parents (Pedro-Carroll, 2005). This chapter examined the practice of group play therapy with children affected by divorce from a Jungian perspective. The Jungian group intervention permits children the opportunity to self-heal through psychoeducation, individual artwork, group encouragement, and finally, parent integration towards the end of the 4-month format. At their disposal, play therapists have a bevy of evidence-based and evidence-informed divorce interventions to support children's mental health. This chapter's authors provided an original intervention of Jungian group play therapy as a potentially beneficial modality to support vulnerable children in their, at times, scary, but hopefully triumphant, post-divorce mental health adjustment.

Appendix

Archetypal Education Instructions for Group Work with Children

A. Rationale: Archetypal education cultivates a child's creativity and inner fantasy life and guides them through the layers of their own inscapes by grounding them through the basic elements and linking these elements to their feelings associated with familial dynamics/divorce. This activity is a vehicle to assist children in developing coping skills following a divorce.

B. Goal: To deepen the child's experience in group counseling by stimulating and involving the child creatively by allowing him to develop and reconnect to a personal response to essential, archetypal elements (Earth, Fire, Water, Wind) in his life.

C. Materials: Construction paper or plain white sheets of paper (preferably larger than standard 8 x 11), markers, colored pencils, paint, paintbrushes, cups of water, different colors of glitter (red, yellow, blue, green), and glue.

D. Procedure: Have the children close their eyes and begin taking deep breaths. Possibly do some muscle relaxation techniques to release any tension. After 2–3 minutes, with soft music playing in the background, produce relaxation, and guided imagery exercise. Focus on one or more of the archetypal elements by saying things like, "You've had experiences with Earth. Imagine you're in the desert. Look around you. See the arid sand. Listen to the sounds. How does your skin feel? Now imagine you're in the jungle. What animals do you see?" Or for Water, you may say things like, "Imagine the feeling of rain falling down upon you. Think about the freshwater running and gurgling in the river. Can you imagine yourself there? Can you see anything in the water? Think of all the images of water as you breathe in and out slowly." Or for Fire, "What does fire look like? Think about the fire. How does it help you? Have you ever seen a fire get out of control?" After the guided imagery portion is completed, have the children draw and project the images they saw in their minds onto paper. The counselor should be in complete silence as the children produce their artwork. If they seek prompting or approval, simply comment, "I can see you are placing a lot of effort into your artwork: thank you." Process the artwork by connecting the images with feelings in their life. How can they gain mastery of these feelings? Which images are calming? Which images express fiery feelings? Accept all interpretations by the group, as the artwork provides the counselor with a deeper understanding of the children and some insights into their psychological state following the divorce.

References

Amato, P. R. (2000). The consequences of divorce for adults and children. *Journal of Marriage and the Family*, 62, 1269–1287. doi:10.1111/j.1741-3737.2000.01269.x.

Baker, A. & Andre, K. (2018). *Getting through my parents' divorce*. Instant Help Books.

Bernet, W. (2020). Parental alienation and misinformation proliferation. *Family Court Review*, 58(2), 293–307. doi:10.1111/fcre.12473.

Bludon-Nash, J. & Schaefer, C. E. (2011). Play therapy: Basics concepts and practices. In C. E. Schaefer (Ed.), *Foundations of play therapy*, (2nd ed. pp. 3–13). John Wiley & Sons.

Chambers, J. (2017). The neurobiology of attachment: From infancy to clinical outcomes. *Psychodynamic Psychiatry*, 45(4), 542–563. doi:10.1521/pdps.2017.45.4.542.

Connolly, M. E. & Green, E. J. (2009). Evidence-based counseling interventions with children of divorce: Implications for elementary school counselors. *Journal of School Counseling*, 7(26), 1–37. doi:212034.

Davies, P. T. & Woitach, M. J. (2008). Children's emotional security in the interparental relationship. *Current Directions in Psychological Science*, 17(4), 269–274. doi:10.1111%2Fj.1467-8721.2008.00588.x.

DeLucia-Waack, J. L. (2006). *Leading psychoeducational groups for children/adolescents*. Sage.

Fidler, B. J. & Ward, P. (2017). Clinical decision-making in parent-child contact problem cases: Tailoring the intervention to the family's needs. In A. M. Judge & R. M. Deutsch (Eds.), *Overcoming parent-child contact problems: Family-based interventions for resistance, rejection, and alienation* (pp. 13–62). Oxford University Press.

Gabbard, G. O. (2017). *Psychodynamic psychiatry in clinical practice*. American Psychiatric Association Publishing.

Green, E. J. (2011). Jungian analytical play therapy. In C. Schaefer (Ed.), *Foundations of play therapy* (2nd ed. pp. 84–100). John Wiley & Sons.

Green, E. J. (2014). *The handbook of Jungian play therapy with children and adolescents*. Johns Hopkins University Press.

Green, E. J. & Myrick, A. C. (2014). Treating complex trauma in adolescents: A phase-based, integrative approach for play therapists. *International Journal of Play Therapy*, 23(3), 131–145. doi:10.1037/a0036679.

Green, E., Myrick, A., & Stephens, R. (2019). Play therapy with children and families affected by conflictual divorce. *Playground*, 4(2), 12–19. doi:10.546xu/09342.

Hetherington, E. M. (2005). Divorce and the adjustment of children. *Pediatrics in Review*, 26(5), 163–169. doi:10.1542/pir.26-5-163.

Judge, A. M. & Bailey, R. (2017). More than words: The use of experiential therapies in the treatment of families with parent-child contact problems and parental alienation. In A. M. Judge & R. M. Deutsch (Eds.), *Overcoming parent-child contact problems*. (pp. 91–106). Oxford University Press.

Pedro-Carroll, J. L. (2005). Fostering resilience in the aftermath of divorce: The role of evidence-based programs for children. *Family Court Review*, 43(1), 52–64. doi:10.1111/j.1744-1617.2005.00007.x.

Poli, C. F., Molgora, S., Marzotto, C., Facchin, F., & Cyr, F. (2017). Group interventions for children having separated parents. *Journal of Divorce & Remarriage*, 58(8), 559–583. https://psycnet.apa.org/doi/10.1080/10502556.2017.1345243.

Pollet, S. L. (2009). A nationwide survey of programs for children of divorcing and separating parents. *Family Court Review*, 47, 523–543. doi:10.1111/j.1744-1617.2009.01271.x.

Rosenberg A. B. (2011). Divorce-stress-adjustment perspective. In S. Goldstein & J. A. Naglieri (Eds.), *Encyclopedia of child behavior and development* (pp. 87–90). Springer. doi:10.1007/978-0-387-79061-9_876.

Sandler, I., Miles, J., Cookston, J., & Braver, S. (2008). Effects of father and mother parenting on children's mental health in high and low conflict divorces. *Family Court Review*, 46(2), 282–296. doi:10.1111/j.1744-1617.2008.00201.x.

Shedler, J. (2010). The efficacy of psychodynamic therapy. *American Psychologist*, 65(2), 98–109. doi:10.1037/a0018378.

van der Kolk, B. (2014). *The body keeps the score: Brain, mind, and body in the healing of trauma*. Viking.

Yalom, I. D. & Leszcz, M. (2005). *The theory and practice of group psychotherapy* (5th ed.). Basic Books.

15 Play Therapy Group Work with Sexually Abused Children

Sueann Kenney-Noziska

According to the United States' current statistics, childhood sexual abuse is estimated to impact approximately 1 in 10 children before their 18th birthday (Townsend & Rheingold, 2013). Estimates may even be higher as low disclosure rates make it difficult to determine a precise number of victims. The impact and sequalae of childhood sexual abuse cannot be underestimated. Without intervention and treatment, the prognosis for victims is poor and may result in impaired functioning across settings. This may include such things as mental health issues, medical problems, social problems, and substance abuse issues, among others.

That being said, effective treatments for childhood trauma, including childhood sexual abuse, have evolved throughout the years and have resulted in improved outcomes for those who have suffered sexual harm at the hands of others. When providing treatment to victims of childhood sexual abuse, multimodal treatment involving individual, group, and family therapy is recommended (Lowenstein & Freeman, 2012). As a means to that end, this chapter will focus on the exploration of play therapy group work for victims of childhood sexual abuse. An integrative, trauma-focused group play therapy approach will be explored with an emphasis on utilizing a variety of play-based interventions. Included in this treatment is an integration of play therapy, group therapy, and trauma-focused core treatment components which are clinically recommended by the National Child Traumatic Stress Network (2020). This is not a manualized group play therapy program, rather a demonstration of ways to integrate tenants of group play therapy within a clinical framework of childhood sexual abuse and trauma-focused elements.

Brief Overview of Childhood Sexual Abuse

Childhood sexual abuse encompasses both contact offenses (for example, fondling of the genitalia, oral copulation, and/or penetration) and noncontact offenses (including voyeurism, online sexual exploitation, and exposure to pornography). It is well-known within the clinical community that sexual victimization can be perpetrated in both intra- and extra-familial contexts

DOI: 10.4324/9781003094531-15

(Townsend & Rheingold, 2013). Intrafamilial childhood sexual abuse impacts the entire family system and there are many barriers for disclosure. These barriers include the close relationship between victim and offender, disbelief by family members, loyalty conflicts, and fear the abuser will get in trouble. There tends to be an increase in disclosure of childhood sexual abuse for older children and adolescents. Likewise, females are more likely to disclose sexual abuse when compared to male victims. Overall, it is believed that only 30% (or less) of all cases of childhood sexual abuse are disclosed in childhood (Tracy, 2012). Intrafamilial childhood sexual abuse is further complicated when there is visitation and reunification of the offender back into the family system.

Interdisciplinary work required for reconciliation and/or reunification include trauma-focused treatment for the victim, sex offender treatment for the perpetrator with a provider specifically trained in sex offending treatment, and involvement of the non-offending caregiver in the offender's treatment. Reparation, reconciliation, and ultimate reunification is *only* conducted if it is in the best interest of the victim. If at any point, reparation, reconciliation, and/or reunification does not appear to be in the victim's best interest, this piece of clinical work is immediately terminated. Typically, this is a team decision with the overarching guiding principle being the child's best interest. A thorough discussion surrounding the mechanisms of reunification post childhood sexual abuse is beyond the scope of this chapter. However, the reader must be aware of the interdisciplinary work of such processes.

Extrafamilial childhood sexual abuse involves perpetration by someone who is in a close role in the child's life but who is outside the family system. Examples include, but are not limited to, teachers, babysitters, coaches, church leaders, and neighbors. As is true with intrafamilial childhood sexual abuse, extrafamilial sexual abuse involves an age differential and frequently involves the perpetrator being in a position of power and/or authority over the victim. Although the negative impact of extrafamilial childhood sexual abuse may mirror that of intrafamilial sexual abuse, the family loyalty conflict is less of a factor and reunification typically does not occur.

The consequences of sexual abuse are well-documented, multifaceted, and complex. Childhood sexual abuse is recognized as a nonspecific risk factor which, in conjunction with other variables, can lead to a variety of struggles for victims (Kenney-Noziska, 2019b). These variables include such things as the relationship between the victim and perpetrator, preexisting mental health issues, family dynamics, and the manner in which the disclosure is handled. These variables can create pathways for psychiatric disorders, substance abuse, eating disorders, and a variety of other struggles for victims. Childhood sexual abuse is linked to many adverse outcomes including mental health issues, physical health problems, and struggles with social, sexual, and interpersonal functioning (Benuto & O'Donohue, 2015; Cashmore & Shackel, 2013; Chen et al., 2010; Conte &

Vaughan-Eden, 2018; Goodyear-Brown, 2012; Lalor & McElvaney, 2010; Trask et al., 2011). Conte and Vaughan-Eden (2018) postulate that a majority of mental health problems and multiple adverse social conditions can be linked to sexual abuse in childhood. Such adverse social conditions can include being revictimized, having struggles maintaining healthy boundaries with others, and low self-esteem. As often seen in clinical settings, victims of childhood sexual abuse can be revictimized in other ways in their future. Subsequently, it is paramount research begins to delve into these mechanisms to undo the cycle of violence and abuse. Research in this area would increase understanding as to why sexual abuse tends to occur in a family system across generations and may highlight targets for intervention and prevention to break this cycle.

Systematic reviews by Chen et al. (2010) and Trask et al. (2011) suggest a connection between sexual abuse in childhood and depression, posttraumatic stress disorder (PTSD), eating disorders, internalizing symptoms, externalizing problems, sexual revictimization, regressed behaviors, suicide attempts, and substance abuse (Kenney-Noziska, 2019b). The most common negative outcomes found in victims of childhood sexual abuse include childhood and adult onset of PTSD symptoms such as intrusion, avoidance, and hyperarousal. This also includes externalizing issues such as regression, aggression, emotional reactivity, defiance, self-injurious behaviors. Furthermore, internalizing problems (i.e., guilt, low self-esteem, withdrawal, somatic complaints, anxiety) are also common (Trask et al., 2011). In addition, research has found (Cashmore & Shackel, 2013) an overall association between childhood sexual abuse and depression, alcohol abuse, substance abuse as well as specific gender-related risk factors of increased eating disorders for women survivors and anxiety-related disorders for male survivors. A systematic review and meta-analysis conducted by Chen et al. (2010) found an association between a history of childhood sexual abuse and several somatic disorders. Certainly, the negative impact of childhood sexual abuse should not be minimized or discounted.

Although childhood sexual abuse has well-documented deleterious effects, it is important to note that not all victims of sexual abuse experience difficulties that require clinical intervention. According to Domhardt et al. (2015), the percentage of childhood sexual abuse survivors found to have a normal level of functioning post sexual abuse ranges from 10% to 53%. In other words, there is a percentage of victims who do not experience clinical levels of posttraumatic symptoms. Subsequently, resiliency and protective factors are important to consider when conceptualizing cases of sexual abuse. Protective factors with the best empirical support for victims of childhood sexual abuse include education, interpersonal and emotional competence, control beliefs, active coping, optimism, social attachment, external attribution of blame, and, most importantly, support from the family and the wider social environment (Domhardt et al., 2015).

Research and Theory of Play Therapy Group Work with Victims of Childhood Sexual Abuse

Both group therapy and individual psychotherapy have been shown to improve psychological symptoms among sexual abuse survivors (Chen et al., 2010). However, according to Yalom and Leszcz (2005), adding group therapy as part of the therapeutic services for victims of sexual abuse may provide benefits beyond individual therapy. These include a reduction in isolation, a decrease in stigmatization, and an increase in support. Play therapy group work with child victims of sexual abuse reduces the isolation and stigmatization commonly experienced in the trauma of their experience. Group play therapy offers unique advantages including universality, vicarious learning, risk-taking, catharsis, and enhancement of interpersonal skills (Lowenstein & Freeman, 2012). For those who have experienced sexual abuse, the benefit of universality can be enormous (Yalom & Leszcz, 2005). It may be in the group setting that victims encounter others who have experienced sexual abuse and may begin to realize that they are truly not alone and are not "damaged". This shared learning experience of universality can be essential in reducing shame, stigma, and self-blame. Additionally, play therapy group work offers an efficient approach for treatment of childhood sexual abuse as it allows for multiple children to be treated concurrently.

Group play therapy may benefit victims of childhood sexual abuse of all ages, although it may look different across the lifespan. For youth, there is quantitative and qualitative support for a wide variety of group therapy modalities and interventions. The use of Activity Group Therapy (AGT) with adolescents (Sweeney et al., 2014) allows time and a safe space for a variety of crafts and games. An example would be having clients completed a "Who am I?" collage to reflect their self-perception. There is also support for expressive arts groups (Gil, 2011; 2017) for children who have experienced abuse and neglect. In this approach, expressive arts are used to process unconscious material related to the child's sexual abuse and provides an outlet for expression.

A play-based group curriculum for children ages 7–12 years (Lowenstein & Freeman, 2012) has also been delineated to provide psychoeducation, emotional expression, and coping strategies in a group format for victims of childhood sexual abuse. This type of group utilizes a primarily psychoeducational, skill-building group format that integrates play-based and expressive arts interventions. Furthermore, game-based cognitive-behavioral therapy in a group format (Springer & Misurell, 2010) emphasizes games to address components of sexual victimization by integrating components of CBT for trauma with structured play therapy. This group also includes a parallel education for the non-offending caregivers who participate in concurrent group sessions. According to Hiller, Springer, Misurell, Kranzler, and Rizvi (2016), using GB-CBT results in improvement in both internalizing and externalizing symptoms, a reduction in sexually inappropriate behaviors, and improved personal safety skills across demographic backgrounds and varied abuse histories. Similarly, group treatment with young sexually abused children has support for use with victims of childhood sexual abuse (Gallo-Lopez, 2006). This program includes using puppet interviews for projection as well as drama therapy with an emphasis on process versus product. For specific details about these protocols, please refer to the original publications.

When utilizing group play therapy for sexually abused preschool children, groups may be coed, shorter in duration, and smaller in terms of the number of group members (Jones, 2002). Less directive groups may be more developmentally appropriate for preschool children and facilitating a concurrent nonoffending parent group is standard. According to Jones (2002), typical play behaviors exhibited by sexually abused preschoolers include: aggression, withdrawal, hypervigilance, sexual behaviors, abuse reenactment, dissociation, regressive-nurturing behaviors, conflict, and boundary problems. Therapists must be mindful of these possible behaviors and be prepared to respond therapeutically. For example, with aggression, Jones (2002) recommends reflecting the feeling, reflecting the meaning behind the feeling, and setting a therapeutic limit. For details on intervening in these types of behaviors, the reader is referred to Jones (2002).

As with other treatment modalities, group composition and structure are key considerations (Sweeney et al., 2014). For victims of childhood sexual abuse, group therapy appears to work best when groups are composed of children of the same gender and close in age (Lowenstein & Freeman, 2012). Group format may be closed (i.e., single cohort) or open (i.e., fluid membership). There are pros and cons to both formats. A closed group provides the foundation for strong cohesion among the cohort; however, this may also result in a waiting list and delayed services for other children. The open group format may minimize wait time but planning group sessions may prove to be a challenge as group members will be at different stages of treatment. An open group format allows victims quicker access to treatment and the possibility of seasoned group members being far enough along in treatment to provide needed support for the new group members.

Group rituals are typical for therapeutic groups. In group play therapy for victims of childhood sexual abuse, a common structure is an opening ritual, a trauma-focused play therapy activity/intervention, and a closing ritual. This can create a solid, clinically-sound 45-minute group session. Opening rituals can include creating a creed for the group which is read at the beginning of each session, sharing feelings, or a brief check-in with each group member at the beginning of each session. Closing rituals can include summarizing the therapeutic concept emphasized in the trauma-focused play therapy intervention, reviewing what was learned, or having a small snack.

There is evidence for the effectiveness of play therapy with various presenting problems (Ray & McCullough, 2016) and research which suggests group play therapy can be an effective intervention for a variety of problems (Sweeney et al., 2014). For childhood sexual abuse and other types of childhood adversity, trauma-focused interventions have the most support for treatment. As such, trauma-focused, play-based interventions appear best suited for group play therapy with victims of childhood sexual abuse. This includes a wide range of play therapy interventions such as play-based techniques, activity-based approaches, puppet play, sand tray, game-based interventions, and expressive arts therapy. For example, facilitating emotional expression secondary to childhood sexual abuse may be facilitated with the play-based intervention Feelings Tic-Tac-Toe (Lowenstein, 1999) in which feelings related to the sexual abuse are identified and processed in the group setting. For psychoeducation related to childhood sexual abuse, *The Sexual Abuse Game* from Paper Dolls and Paper Airplanes (Crisci et al., 1998), may serve useful. This therapeutic, play-based intervention provides a foundation for exploring reactions to trauma, discussing dynamics of CSA, and dispelling misperceptions. As the clinical profiles of sexual victims are heterogenous, an integrative approach to group play therapy may be best suited for sexual abuse treatment (Gil, 2006; Gil, 2011; Gil, 2017; Kenney-Noziska, 2019a; Kenney-Noziska, 2019b). Such an approach involves the use of the blending of nondirective and directive interventions based within solid theory. Using the core components of evidenced based treatment as described by the NCTCS (2020) should serve as the guide for choosing the play therapy or expressive intervention. This process is driven by the therapeutic needs of the group members.

As defined by the National Child Traumatic Stress Network (2020), intervention objectives for trauma treatment include: psychoeducation about trauma reminders and loss reminders, psychoeducation about post-traumatic stress reactions and grief reactions, teaching emotional regulation skills, constructing a trauma narrative, and teaching safety skills. Psychoeducation and emotional regulation skills serve to strengthen coping skills. Constructing a trauma narrative is geared toward reducing posttraumatic stress reactions. Whereas safety skills, such as healthy boundaries and learning "red flags" of abuse, serve to promote interpersonal safety and reduce the likelihood of future victimization. With the exception of trauma narratives, which is not done in a group setting as it may result in vicarious trauma for group members, these can serve as important intervention targets for group play therapy.

Group Example/Intervention

This case example is a clinical compilation of group play therapy for a group of adolescent females who were enrolled in middle school and had experienced childhood sexual abuse at the hands of a relative, also known as intrafamilial sexual abuse. The group therapy format consists of beginning group by reading the group creed and sharing feelings for the day. This is followed by a trauma-focused play therapy intervention which targets a specific intervention objective as delineated by National Child Traumatic Stress Network (2020). For example, if the group session is focused on facilitating emotional identification and expression secondary to childhood sexual abuse, the game *Revealing Your Feelings* (Kenney-Noziska, 2008), an intervention that requires players to identify and explore feelings related to sexual abuse while revealing emotions using Crayola^{TM} Color Switchers (markers that change color), may be utilized. The last several minutes of group is snack time. Each group session is 45 minutes in length.

Savannah is a 12-year-old female with a history of childhood sexual abuse at the hands of her stepfather. She is receiving individual therapy by a community provider and was referred to the sexual abuse group therapy program as an adjunct service. She presents with posttraumatic symptoms which negatively impact her functioning across settings. She has clinical levels of anxiety, depression, and overall posttraumatic stress on the Trauma Symptom Checklist for Children (TSCC) rating scale and struggles with anxiety, nightmares, social withdrawal, and intrusive recollections of the sexual abuse. Savannah joins the middle school group which consists of four other girls: Becky, Annie, Addison, and Leah. For Savannah's first session, the intervention *Ice Breaker* (Kenney-Noziska, 2008) was used to build group rapport and establish the therapeutic relationship. In this technique, players share information about themselves based on the color of sticker on the underside of the ice cubes. Annie shared a love for drawing and playing volleyball. Addison and Leah shared similar interests and a brief exploration of these commonalities occurred. One area of commonality processed during the activity was the fact that all of the girls had a history of childhood sexual abuse. This served as a foundation to explore the isolation and stigma inherent in sexual trauma. Savannah shared feelings of isolation and a belief that she was the only child with a history of childhood sexual abuse prior to attending group. However, after meeting the other group members, she verbalized an understanding that she is not alone.

Psychoeducation to help Savannah and the other group members understand the concept and impact of sexual abuse was integrated throughout treatment and occurred frequently at the onset of therapy. Therapeutic games from *Paper Dolls and Paper Airplanes* (Crisci et al., 1998) including *The Sexual Abuse Game* and *Myth & Facts*, provided a foundation for exploring reactions to trauma, discussing dynamics of sexual abuse, and dispelling misperceptions of the role of the victim and perpetrator. *The Sexual Abuse Game* (Crisci et al., 1998) includes feeling, learning, and telling cards whereby perceptions, dynamics, and triggers related to sexual abuse were processed. Savannah identified a belief that she is responsible for the sexual abuse she experienced as she did not say "no" and did not stop it from occurring. She also processed feelings of sadness and confusion as to why the sexual abuse happened and why it happened to her. Becky, another group member, offered the idea that Savannah may never know the answers to those questions but, nevertheless, healing was possible.

The next several sessions focused on emotional regulation skills. *Feeling Faces* (Crisci et al., 1998) was used to process feelings specific to childhood sexual abuse. The activity allows group members to complete sentences pertaining to childhood sexual abuse with various emotions. Savannah received support from other group members as she shared feelings of guilt and embarrassment. Group members that experienced similar emotions joined with Savannah and echoed her feelings. During a following session, the intervention *On a Scale of 1 to 10* (S. Kenney-Noziska, personal communication, December 29, 2020) was utilized to explore feelings on a deeper level. During this intervention, group members take turns ranking feelings related to childhood sexual abuse on a scale of intensity from 1 (rarely experience) to 10 (constantly experience). Savannah ranked the feeling "hopeful" as a 2. She discussed feeling as if things were too much and would never get better. Leah, a fellow group member, was able to empathize with feeling hopeless when she first began the group as well but, with therapy and support, discussed being hopeful for her future. This exchange appeared to provide Savannah a sense of relief.

Several play therapy techniques were used to facilitate the development of use of healthy coping strategies including *Lemon Squeezies* (Mellenthin, 2018), a full body relaxation technique involving guided imagery. As this activity was processed, Savannah shared trouble sleeping at night as the sexual abuse would occur while she was in bed. Two other group members were able to identify similar experiences and, from that foundation, the bedtime/nighttime issues were normalized, and the group processed sleep hygiene routines in an attempt to improve sleep patterns. Additionally, *Positive and Negative Thinking* (Kenney-Noziska, 2008) was used to address cognitive coping skills with an emphasis on understanding the difference between general positive and negative cognitions. During the clinical intervention, group members determine whether a statement is a positive statement or a negative statement, then reads the statement using the tone of voice and facial expression communicating the statement as identified and places the card in the pile as either positive or negative. This provided a foundation to explore childhood sexual abuse-specific cognitions. As a group member processed feeling guilty about the childhood sexual abuse for not telling sooner, Savannah shared that when she disclosed her childhood sexual abuse to her mother, her mother's response was, "Why didn't you tell me sooner?". The therapist was able to normalize this reaction and discussed the process nonoffending parents/caregivers go through as they figure out how to maneuver the nuances of sexual abuse. This can include initial disbelief, nonsupport, and shock and may result in the nonoffending caregiver needing their own therapy to work through these stages to reach a point where they can believe, support, and protect the victim.

The next area of focus for the group was processing the dynamics of childhood sexual abuse. *The Spider and the Fly: Bibliotherapy for Understanding Perpetrators* (Cavett, 2010) was used to explore enticement strategies utilized by offenders. This intervention explores enticement strategies utilized by sex offenders and provides a baseline from which group members may begin to identify the strategies used by their particular offender. As a follow-up to this intervention, *Types of Abusers* (Crisci et al., 1998) provided the foundation for differentiating between enticement strategies for the nice abuser, mean abuser, sad abuser, lying abuser, sneaky abuser, and blaming abuser. Similar to *The Spider and the Fly* noted above, this intervention breaks offender enticement strategies into categories and provides a framework for group members to process the "tricks" used by their abusers. In conjunction with her fellow group members, Savannah was able to process that her stepfather was a "nice abuser" who used strategies of kindness to make her trust him and not disclose the abuse that had taken place. Specifically, Savannah shared receiving extra privileges and gifts that her siblings did not receive.

Community Crown (Goodyear-Brown, 2002) was used to identify a post-childhood sexual abuse support system. In this activity, Savannah identified people who believe and support her disclosure of sexual abuse. She drew her mother as half a person and shared with the group that she was unsure how much belief and support she received from her mother. She further processed this by sharing a belief that her mother, in part, blames Savannah for the abuse that took place in their home. As she shared this, Savannah was joined by Addison, a fellow group member who experiences a similar belief. Noticeable on Savannah's Community Crown was "group members". Savannah teared up as she heartfeltly processed how much support she received from her fellow group members and how she was unsure of where she would be in her healing process without them.

As termination neared, we explored safety and coping strategies to utilize post-termination. *A Safe Place for a Stone* (Makin, 2000) allowed Savannah to create a safe space via the metaphor of an art scene made to give the "stone" (i.e., the self) a safe space for healing. Savannah identified the group as a "safe space" and expressed sadness for "graduating" from group therapy and shared that she will miss the group members' support. Following this activity, the next group therapy session the *Coping Collage* (Goodyear-Brown, 2010) was implemented, whereby Savannah and her fellow group members created a collage of their favorite things and positive upcoming events to assist in maintaining a sense of positive anticipation during stressful times.

Group play therapy for Savannah ended with an open-door option, allowing for follow-up, check-up, or check-in sessions as needed posttreatment. This type of termination is especially important for victims of childhood sexual abuse, as it is suggested that adolescent and adult milestones may result in issues and struggles related to sexual abuse resurfacing (Hindman, 1989). At last contact, Savannah was doing well.

Conclusion

A multimodal approach to treating childhood sexual abuse, including a combination of individual, group, and family therapy, may obtain optimal results (Lowenstein & Freeman, 2012). Group work is an important component of that multimodal treatment. Play therapy group work can be a valuable component for addressing posttraumatic suffering secondary to childhood sexual abuse and provides a developmentally sensitive treatment approach for children and adolescents. While individual and family therapy can be helpful for sexually abused children, there are unique advantages of group play therapy including reduced isolation and stigmatization (Lowenstein & Freeman, 2012). Indeed, as asserted by Yalom and Leszcz (2005), group therapy is a potentially potent modality with substantial benefits for participants.

References

Benuto, L. E. & O'Donohue, W. (2015). Treatment of sexually abused children: A review and synthesis of recent meta-analyses. *Children and Youth Services Review*, 56, 52–56.

Cashmore, J. & Shackel, R. (2013, January). The long-term effects of child sexual abuse (Child Family Community Australia Paper 11). *Australian Institute of Family Studies*. https://aifs.gov.au/cfca/sites/default/files/cfca/pubs/papers/a143161/cfca11.pdf.

Cavett, A. M. (2010). *Structured play-based interventions for engaging children and adolescents in therapy*. Infinity Publishing.

Chen, L. P., Murad, M. H., Paras, M. L., Colbenson, K. M., Sattler, A. L., Goranson, E. N., Elamin, M. B., Seime, R. J., Shinozakig, G., Prokon, L. Z., & Zirakzadeh, A. (2010). Impact of child sexual abuse and lifetime diagnosis of psychiatric disorders: Systematic review and meta-analysis. *Mayo Clinical Proceedings*, 85(7), 618–629.

Conte, J. R. & Vaughan-Eden, V. (2018). Child sexual abuse. In J. B. Klika & J. R. Conte (Eds.), *The APSAC handbook on child maltreatment* (4th ed., pp. 95–110). Sage.

Crisci, G., Lay, M., & Lowenstein, L. (1998). *Paper dolls and paper airplanes: Therapeutic activities for sexually traumatized children*. Kidsrights.

Domhardt, M., Münzer, A., Feget, J. M., & Gikdbeck, L. (2015). Resilience in survivors of child sexual abuse: A systematic review of the literature. *Trauma, Violence & Abuse*, 16(4), 476–493.

Gallo-Lopez, L. (2006). A creative play therapy approach to the group treatment of young sexually abused children. In Kaduson, H. & Schaefer, C. E. (Eds.), *Short term play therapy for children* (2nd ed.) (pp. 245–272). Guilford.

Gil, E. (2006). *Helping abused and traumatized children: Integrating directive and nondirective approaches.* Guilford Press.

Gil, E. (2011). *Working with children to heal interpersonal trauma: The power of play.* Guilford Press.

Gil, E. (2017). *Posttraumatic play in children: What clinicians need to know.* Guilford Press.

Goodyear-Brown, P. (2002). *Digging for buried treasure: 52 prop-based play therapy interventions for treating the problems of childhood.* Sundog Publishing.

Goodyear-Brown, P. (2010). *Play therapy with traumatized children: A prescriptive approach.* Wiley & Sons.

Goodyear-Brown, P. (Ed.) (2012). *Handbook of childhood sexual abuse: Identification, assessment, and treatment.* Wiley & Sons, Inc.

Hiller, A., Springer, C., Misurell, J., Kranzler, A., & Rizvi, S. (2016). Predictors of group treatment outcomes for child sexual abuse: An investigation of the role of demographic and abuse characteristics. *Child Abuse Review*, 25(2), 102–114. https://cmps-ezproxy.mnu.edu:2299/10.1002/car.2343.

Hindman, J. (1989). *Just before dawn: From the shadows of tradition to new reflections in trauma assessment and treatment for sexual victimization.* Alexandria Associates.

Jones, K. D. (2002). Group play therapy with sexually abused preschool children: Group behaviors and interventions. *Journal for Specialists in Group Work*, 27(4), 377–389. https://cmps-ezproxy.mnu.edu:2299/10.1080/714860200.

Kenney-Noziska, S. (2008). *Techniques-techniques-techniques: Play-based activities for children, adolescents, and families.* Infinity Publishing.

Kenney-Noziska, S. (2019a). Integrating directive and posttraumatic play therapy to address childhood trauma. *Play Therapy Magazine*, 14(2), 12–15.

Kenney-Noziska, S. (2019b). Therapeutic games for sexually abused children. In Schaefer, C. E. & Stone, J. (Eds.), *Game Play* (3rd ed.). Wiley and Sons.

Lalor, K. & McElvaney, R. (2010). Child sexual abuse, links to later sexual exploitation/high risk sexual behavior, and prevention/treatment programmes. *Trauma, Violence, and Abuse*, 11, 159–177.

Lowenstein, L. (1999). *Creative interventions for troubled children and youth.* Champion Press.

Lowenstein, L. & Freeman, R. C. (2012). Group therapy with sexually abused children. In Goodyear-Brown, P. (Ed.) (2012). *Handbook of childhood sexual abuse: Identification, assessment, and treatment.* John Wiley & Sons, Inc.

Makin, S. R. (2000). *Therapeutic art directives and resources: Activities and initiatives for individuals and groups.* Jessica Kingsley Publisher.

Mellenthin, C. (2018). *Play Therapy: Engaging and powerful techniques for the treatment of childhood disorders.* Pesi Publishing.

National Child Traumatic Stress Network. (2020). *Core components of trauma-informed interventions.* Retrieved from www.nctsn.org/treatments-and-practices/trauma-treatments/overview.

Ray, D. C. & McCullough, R. (2016). *Evidence-based practice statement: Play therapy (Research report).* Association for Play Therapy. www.a4pt.org/?page=EvidenceBased.

Springer, C. & Misurell, J. R. (2010). Game-based cognitive-behavioral therapy (GB-CBT): An innovative group treatment program for children who have been sexually abused. *Journal of Child and Adolescent Trauma, 3,* 163–180. doi:10.1080/19361521.2010.491506.

Sweeney, D. S., Baggerly, J. N., & Ray, D. C. (2014). *Group play therapy: A dynamic approach.* Routledge.

Townsend, C. & Rheingold, A. A. (2013). *Estimating a child sexual abuse prevalence rate for practitioners: A review of child sexual abuse prevalence studies.* Darkness2-Light. www.d2l.org/wp-content/uploads/2017/02/PREVALENCE-RATE-WHITE-PAPER-D2L.pdf.

Tracy, N. (2012, July 23). *Child Sexual Abuse Statistics, HealthyPlace.* Retrieved on 2020, December 6 from www.healthyplace.com/abuse/child-sexual-abuse/child-sexual-abuse-statistics.

Trask, E., Walsh, K., & DiLillo, D. (2011). Treatment effects for common outcomes of child sexual abuse: A current meta-analysis. *Aggression and Violent Behavior, 16,* 6–19.

Yalom, I. D. & Leszcz, M. (2005). *The theory and practice of group psychotherapy* (5th ed.). Basic Books.

16 Play Based Group Retreat for Adoptive Families

Theresa Fraser

Group therapy enables group members to take on roles to support and strengthen each other as well as impact the thoughts, feelings, attitudes, and potential behaviors (of self and others). Where long-term therapy can occur over months, short-term group therapy is focused and structured. Directive activities can be connected to specific goals that all members wish to address (Center for Substance Abuse Treatment, 1999). This chapter reviews a short intensive multifamily group therapy experience that incorporates the therapeutic powers of play (Schaefer & Drewes, 2013) in order to support adoptive families and their chosen children.

Children who are removed from their biological families and later placed in a foster or adoptive family require their needs to be viewed from an attachment lens. Dr. John Bowlby first published the importance of an infant being cared for by an emotionally sensitive and attuned caregiver (1988). Mary Ainsworth (1913–1999), built on this seminal work underscoring the importance of creating a safe base for children by researching the separation and reunion of parent and child. According to Kerr and Cossar (2014) a parent/child safe base is important for children to return to particularly in response to stress inducing experiences.

Selwyn, Wijedasa, and Meakings (2016) shared that up to 74% of children who are adopted have experienced adverse childhood experiences related to 1) sexual, physical, and/or emotional abuse, 2) exposure to neglect, 3) domestic violence, 4) have perinatal mental health challenges caused by exposure to drugs or alcohol and these experiences typically create attachment disruptions. Additionally, older children who have experienced multiple placement changes can demonstrate subsequent behavioral challenges, and children who have specialized needs such as physical or learning disabilities are also at risk for placement disruption (Fratter, 1991). In a study involving 249 families (who adopted 373 children), it was identified that their post-adoption unmet service needs included counseling, in-home supports, as well as other informal supports. Families shared that these unmet needs perpetuated both disconnection between children and parents, as well as having an overall negative impact on the marriage and family system (Reilly & Platz, 2004). In contemporary times, the majority of adoption supports within

DOI: 10.4324/9781003094531-16

North America have primarily focused on matching, placement, and finalization of adoption. There is growing recognition that post-adoption finalization support is both needed and appreciated by families (Kim & Tucker, 2020), and that this support should include increasing awareness of various available resources (Paine et al., 2020).

It is likely that children who have had no prior experience with a safe base may require specific attachment-based interventions in order to ultimately create and maintain a healthy attachment. Information about attachment and trauma is paramount when parenting a child with adverse childhood experiences. Adoptees who have experienced multiple placement disruptions due to growing up in the child welfare system require caregivers who not only understand trauma and attachment issues, but also how parenting a high needs child can contribute to issues of countertransference. Therefore, assisting adopters to understand the impact of the child's trauma history, developmental needs, and attachment needs is crucial (Felitti et al., 1998). Adverse childhood experiences can also impact brain development (Perry & Szalavitz, 2008) hence, restorative activities and approaches to mediate such development need to underpin trauma-focused parenting. Unfortunately, the need has not been met with the creation of a method/model designed to help children and families with these unique needs.

Brady (2014) states,

> Currently, there is no single evidence-based, post-adoption service model available in the literature. Organizations draw from diverse service and support approaches and tend to tailor post-adoption programs to reflect family needs, existing service delivery systems, and available resources.
>
> (p. 2)

Research Literature Review

Group approaches provide opportunities for social learning, development of an additional support system, networking, and reinforcement for positive change. Being a group member means there is peer support as well as the opportunity to learn new skills. Participants can reflect on intervention outcomes both successful and unsuccessful. These aspects of group treatment can also include multifamily members as group participants.

Multifamily group therapy (MFGT) is a marriage between family and group therapy approaches. A family systems approach combined within a group therapy format can accelerate and enrich the therapeutic process (Hollins, Gritzer, & Okun, 1983). MFGT has been successful for families supporting children with depression (Hellemans, 2011), addiction (Liu et al., 2015), in patient psychiatry programs (Pascoe et al., 2016), and first episode psychosis (Selakovic et al., 2020). MFGT has been identified as a unique treatment modality involving a trained therapist supporting two or more families and utilizing "deliberate, planned psychosocial interventions" that support families to address immediate systemic needs (Thorngren et al., 2002, p. 167). Addressing needs in the community of a small group is not only less costly in regard to therapist time but also provides an opportunity to normalize the family experience. Psychosocial interventions can also include child guidance principles. These interventions can be short-term involving education supports, clinical supports, referrals for basic or material needs, and connecting families to support networks (Brady, 2014).

Although empirical evidence is lacking on the effectiveness of post-adoption services, it is clear adoptive parents want to be engaged in service provision (Barth & Miller, 2000). Engaging in short-term or even one day group experience can provide adoptive families with the opportunity to experience prescriptive interventions such as attachment psychoeducation and trauma-focused parenting approaches that address the varied needs of multiple adoptive families. "Groups tend to promote spontaneity in all clients of all ages and therefore, may increase their participation in play or expressive play experiences (Sweeney et al., 2014, p. 6)". The following intervention examples have been utilized with adoptive families for one day interventions labeled as Adoption Retreat Days.

Group Example Intervention

It is important prior to beginning MFGT the clinician spend time learning about the family's unique adoption narrative to ascertain if they are appropriate for the one-day program. Topics to be discussed include fertility issues, past use of resources, grief process, attachment history, as well as hopes and dreams. This helps to build a therapeutic relationship and safe environment, especially as facilitators establish a non-blaming, non-pathologizing atmosphere for all group members. This is how success is achieved in multi-family psychoeducational programs (Steinglass et al., 2011).

At the beginning of the day camp, the therapist initiates a conversation about confidentiality stressing that stories shared should be honored by practicing respect for privacy for other retreat participants. Therapists who utilize play can identify the most successful activities that will provide all group members with the opportunity to both "observe and synthesize experiences of others in the group including their own family members" (Steinglass et al., 2011, para 18). It has been observed by this author that parents who have positive experiences after attending a family retreat day are more likely to engage in further therapeutic programs, especially if they feel comfortable with the therapist(s) and play-based spaces where intervention occurs.

Morning Activities for Children

The morning is facilitated by two or three staff who are available to support the children's play-based therapeutic activities.

> Play provides an opportunity for children to join with others, to see their world for what it is and has been, to understand it a bit better, to express emotions about what has come their way, and to resolve a new way to survive.
>
> (Riedel, Bowers, & Bowers, 2013, p. 1)

It can be very helpful to have older adolescents or young adults who are also adoptees as support staff and as appropriate, they can share their adoption story.

Morning Theraplay® Integration

Theraplay® helps to adapt some of the internal attachment models that adoptive children develop due to previous experience. The activities are facilitated by therapists that have taken Theraplay® training. These activities support children in feeling both safe and secure while providing the parent with the tools to co-regulate with their children through the very often physical but fun activities (Stock et al., 2016). These attachment-focused activities are categorized under four domains of parent/child interaction: engagement, structure, nurture, and challenge. Table 16.1 provides domain activity examples.

Additionally, the following questions are woven into the morning program about family roles, goals, and activities:

Table 16.1 Theraplay Domain Activity Examples Adapted from Booth and Jernberg (2009)

Engagement – initiates social engagement systems between child and caregiver	Special handshakes, hello song, decorating nails, popping cheeks
Structure – creates safety by setting limits kindly so positive experiences can follow with connection	Stack of hands, row row row your boat, thumb wrestling
Nurture – caregiver supports child to feel cared for	Feeding activities, notices hurts/cuts and puts lotion on them
Challenge – mastery and subsequent confidence building activities	Cotton ball hockey where straws are utilized to blow cotton back and forth at a table or over a line masked with tape on the floor, newspaper punch
Play – joy and bonding	Play is integrated in all dimensions

- What is great about your family?
- What are activities that you do together that are fun?
- Who is the funniest, most reliable, most creative family member, etc.?

These conversations will help the children to participate in afternoon family activities, such as creating a family flag or family cheer based on the identification of familial strengths and unique qualities.

Morning Activities for Parents: Psychoeducation

While the children are engaged in play-based activities, their parents are engaged in psychoeducation activities. These activities assist parents in understanding the impact of early childhood neglect and abuse on brain development and functioning, world view, and ultimately, attachment with primary caregivers. In 2015, Dr. Zill of The Institute for Family Studies identified that adopted children can be impacted by early stress, behavioral genetics, and genetic endowment. Additionally, parents can experience post-adoptive depression (Kappler, 2020) as they adapt to their significant role adjustment.

According to an Ontario, Canada survey of adoption practitioners, parents most often request child guidance specifically on how to manage their child's behaviors, ensuring that they address the needs of other familial members including parents and the marital relationship. Additionally, parents' express interest in finding other support persons who understand adoption-focused attachment parenting (Brady, 2014). Providing psychoeducation gives the opportunity for parents to recognize that they are not the only parents having challenges in their adoption journey. Normalization of these experiences provides a foundation for openness of future clinical interventions.

Lunch Time

Families can bring a dish that represents their culture or is a family or child's favorite to share in a potluck-style luncheon. The retreat sponsors can also purchase a culturally appropriate dish that is kid-friendly such as samosas or pizza. Food, however, should be provided to the children by their parents in order to facilitate bonding and food security. By inviting the parent to plate the food and serve their child, this models how feeding is experienced as nurturing, thereby deepening the parent/child attachment (Rowell, 2012). Lunch time is intended to be a short experience where the family enjoys sharing food without power struggles and where the family experiences repetitive, patterned, relationship, and somatosensory building interactions (Perry & Dobson, 2012).

Afternoon Activity Choices

The afternoon consists of MFGT interventions and play-based activities. These activities encourage the family (parents and children) to communicate common goals and values regarding how they engage together and how they connect with others in the world. It is hoped that as the parents and children engage in these activities, they are enjoying each other's company, fostering attunement and regulation, as well as creating/confirming their family culture. Hughes (2007) refers to this as intersubjectivity, "Parents and children affectively and cognitively present with each other and when the vitality of their states are matched, their cognitive function is focused on the same event or object - their intentions are congruent."

(p. 14).

Family Cheer

A family cheer is created as a testament to the new family's identity such as:

> "We are the Frasers. We like to play. We swim together and read together every single day."

Or

> "We are the Coynes. We try every day to help each other. So there is time left over to play and say, 'I love you'."

Family Sandtray

The family is introduced to sandtray therapy and can utilize any of the available miniatures to create a world in a therapeutic sandtray. An example of this can be the family creating a world that explains the family culture such as what would happen if your family lived in a land with no rules (Fraser, 2010). This activity was created to assist children who have not had safe caregivers to gain insight into a family experience that is safe and secure. Families can also be invited to pick miniatures that represent the personality of family members or a miniature that represents past or current familial cultural stories (Gil, 2016).

Family Flag or Coat of Arms

The family is provided with white broadcloth and crayons or fabric markers. As a family, they can identify their familial strengths and values. The children have already been exposed to these topics by therapists in the morning session. Family members can choose symbols to draw on their flag that represent family strength. If they would rather complete a coat of arms, they can draw the coat of arms on the material and divide it into four quadrants. Each quadrant can represent: a familial belief, shared strength, hope or goal, and favorite shared activities.

After each participating family has finished their activities, they present these outputs to the larger group. This presentation normalizes that adoptive children can experience a sense of belonging and can be cared for by their adoptive parents. With consent, the therapist videotapes this presentation so each family gets a special individualized memento. A family photo can also be taken for the family to have emailed to them after the retreat or a photo booth could be created where family members can obtain immediate photos. They can also receive photos of their flag and/or coat of arms.

Case Example

Mary and Jonah had experienced infertility throughout their 10-year marriage. They were contacted to adopt a sibling group consisting of brothers, aged 9 and 11 years. The children's father had died after the birth of the youngest child. The boy's mother experienced subsequent depression after losing her husband. She ended up getting into a car accident, sustained a back injury, and then required painkillers. She became addicted to opiates and then started to use heroin. She was disconnected from her husband's family once she began her consistent use of substances. Additionally, she grew up in foster care and had no connection with biological family members.

The boys were frequently left alone while the mother was drug seeking. On one occasion, the older sibling attempted to cook for his younger sibling, a kitchen fire occurred, and all the families' belongings were lost. The firemen found the children alone and unsupervised at the age of 7 and 9, and they were subsequently placed in an emergency receiving foster home.

Not long after they were moved to a long-term foster home; this home reminded the boys culturally of their paternal grandparent's home. The children were the only ones placed in this home and they flourished. They enjoyed family activities together, had positive school placements, and were gaining weight from being served nutritious food. Sadly, the foster father died of a heart attack and the foster mother felt unable to provide ongoing foster care to the boys. A parallel process was happening in family court and it became apparent that the judge was more likely to permit the children to be adopted if the children were placed in a "foster to adopt" home where they could experience permanency. Mary and Jonah provided a culturally appropriate home and lived in an affluent neighborhood with wonderful schools. They agreed to become temporary foster parents to the children knowing that once wardship was declared they could begin the adoption trial period.

Once placed, the children's demeanor changed. They demonstrated behaviors not seen by their previous foster mother. They both had difficulty sleeping and would refuse to eat the food provided by their adopted mother, stating that she did not know how to cook like they were used to.

School reports were negative, and the older sibling was sent home often for not listening to authority figures and engaging in aggressive behavior at recess time.

The younger sibling was more open to interactions with Mary. She would read him nighttime stories, but the older brother would complain that she was being annoying and remind his sibling at every opportunity that she was not their mother and that they did not need to listen to her. Mary indicated that she felt helpless and defeated because her sons refused to acknowledge or accept her parental authority.

The boys were much more positive in their interactions with their new dad. They would follow through on expectations when he was home and he verbalized to the therapist that he did not have the same concerns that his wife did. He queried if she was experiencing post-adoptive depression as she was having a difficult time parenting these seemingly easy-going children.

This parenting rift was beginning to negatively affect their marriage. Mary began personal counseling for her symptoms of sleeplessness, constant headaches, fatigue, and feelings of depression. Given Jonah's work schedule, the family could not engage in regular therapy but were open to attending the adoptive family play-based retreat. The children were initially not interested in participating when the play therapists facilitated morning activities. When they saw other children participating in the Theraplay® activities they began to laugh and giggle, especially when they played cotton ball hockey. The younger boy was happy to meet some other adopted children and stated that he did not know any other adopted kids at his school. His older sibling was initially resistant to participating but was eager to hear the story of the program volunteer who was also adopted at the age of 11.

During the morning session, Mary and Jonah were able to verbalize that their adopting journey was not as expected. The couple found themselves in conflict often and they had little time to spend together. Mary verbalized feeling overwhelmed and felt incompetent when she needed to discipline these two boys (one of whom attempted to be physically intimidating to her when her husband is not at home). The other adoptive parents shared that they had some common experiences in navigating their marriage relationships and in disciplining children who do not appear to be impacted by any earned consequences. All parents identified that extended family and friends lacked understanding of the challenge of creating parent/child attachment with children who have had multiple placements and attachment figures. They all wanted to create support systems that would not undermine their parenting attempts but would also help them to build capacity as competent and confident parents.

When the retreat participants came together for lunch, the boys were initially reserved and would not eat anything that their mom had brought to share. The older child attempted to seek out something to eat from one of the morning therapists who redirected him to connect with his mom. He did so begrudgingly but actually ate the food Mary had plated for him.

In the afternoon MFGT session, the boys showed much more interest in being involved, including sharing excitement in making a family cheer and flag. They then created a world using the sandtray. Initially there were no parents or caregivers in the sandtray world, only children until the youngest sibling placed a mother bear in the sandtray. When they took the therapists on a world tour, he proudly shared how the mother bear was protective of the baby animals in the world.

The end of the day came quickly and both boys were not in a hurry to leave. They were happy to take photos of their sandtray world which depicted family activities that the family had already engaged in. They had completed a family flag and coat of arms, both of which chronicled family themes such as eating together, reading together, and having fun together. The clinician observed that there was a lot of eye contact between the parents and the children while they engaged in these activities. The youngest son actually crawled into their mother's lap while the children discussed their flag and coat of arms. While there, he let her stroke his hair. Mary shared at the end of the day that this was a parenting affirming activity for her.

Mary and Jonah engaged in a follow-up session with the clinician and indicated that pursuant to the Adoptive Family Retreat they decided to begin marriage counseling as they both recognized that their own parenting was being impacted by their attachment wounds. After they engaged in these sessions, they requested family Theraplay® sessions. The boys' adoption was finalized fourteen months later. The parents checked in with the therapist five years later and reported the boys were enjoying school and hockey.

Summary

Adoption competent therapists understand that working from a familial perspective will impact the family system holistically, but it also empowers adoptive parents to be the agents of change for their own child(ren). Interventions need to be playful (Schaefer & Drewes, 2013) and integrative (Zarbo et al., 2016), and always focused on supporting the permanency of the family while incorporating community support. According to Brady (2014), these interventions can provide normative support as the child and family move through developmental stages.

Engaging adoptive families in therapy can take many forms including couples therapy, individual therapy, parent coaching, therapeutic groups, and family therapy. Each can contribute to supporting the family in their goal for placement permanency. Short-term interventions such as a one-day group retreat can provide intervention that meets the family where they are, in their moment of need. Family group retreats further support families who cannot engage in long-term services. All families benefit from exposure to other adoptive families and relational play-based interventions. MFGT group retreats can also provide families with the opportunity to see *what might be* with the support of hearing from other families while gaining the support of clinicians and peers who share their experiences and understand the neurobiology of trauma. MFGT retreats open up the possibility for couples, children, or families to engage in additional supportive services given children who have been in foster care and are later adopted are more vulnerable for mental health challenges than children who grow up in biological families (Pinto, 2019).

The hope with a short-term group is that "adoptive children and adoptive families can grow together, heal their traumas, and learn to be more attuned, joyful families" (Webb, 2008, p. 47). If additional supports are needed as a result of pre-existing or subsequent complex needs, families will likely be more amenable to interventions because they have completed a positive therapeutic experience through a one-day group retreat.

References

Barth, R. & Miller, J. (2000). Building effective post-adoption services: What is the empirical foundation? *Family Relations*, 49(4), 447–455. Retrieved December 25, 2020, from www.jstor.org/stable/585840.

Booth, P. B. & Jernberg, A.M. (2009). *Theraplay: Helping parents and children build better relationships through attachment based play* (3rd ed.). Jossey-Bass.

Bowlby J. (1988). *A secure base: Clinical applications of attachment theory.* Routledge.

Brady, E. (2014). *Post adoption support: Recommendations for practitioners and organizations.* Adopt Ontario. www.adoptontario.ca/uploads/File/Post-adoption_ Support_-_Recommendations_for_Practitioners__Organizations-June_2014.pdf.

Center for Substance Abuse Treatment. (1999). *Brief interventions and brief therapies for substance abuse* (Vol. 34). Substance Abuse and Mental Health Services Administration. www.ncbi.nlm.nih.gov/books/NBK64936/.

Felitti, V. J., Anda, R. F., Nordenberg, D., Williamson, D. F., Spitz, A. M., Edwards, V., Koss, M. P., & Marks, J. S. (1998). Relationship of childhood abuse and household dysfunction to many of the leading causes of death in adults. The Adverse Childhood Experiences (ACE) study. *American Journal of Preventive Medicine*, 14(4), 245–258. doi:10.1016/s0749-3797(98)00017–00018.

Fraser, T. (2010). Land of no rules. In L. Lowenstein (Ed.), *Creative family therapy techniques* (pp. 67–70). Champion Press.

Fratter, J., Rowe, J., Sapsford, D., & Thoburn, J. (1991). *Permanent family placement: A decade of experience.* BAAF.

Gil, E. (2016). *Play in family therapy* (2nd ed.). The Guilford Press.

Hellemans, S., De Mol, J., Buysse, A., Eisler, I., Demyttenaere, K., & Lemmens, G. (2011). Therapeutic processes in multi-family groups for major depression: Results of an interpretative phenomenological study. *Journal of Affective Disorders*, 134(1–3), 226–234.

Hollins Gritzer, P. H. & Okun, H. S. (1983) Multiple family group therapy. In Wolman B. B., Stricker G., Framo J., Newirth J. W., Rosenbaum M., & Young H. H. (Eds.), *Handbook of family and marital therapy*. Springer. doi:10.1007/978-1-4684-4442-1_15.

Hughes, D. A. (2007). *Attachment focused family therapy*. W. W. Norton and Co. Incorporated.

Kappler, M. (2020). *Post-adoption depression is a problem we don't talk about enough. Huff Post*. www.huffingtonpost.ca/entry/post-adoption-depression-syndrome_ca_5ec416d3c5b66f94862ef72c.

Kim, J. & Tucker, A. (2020). The inclusive family support model: Facilitating openness for post-adoptive families. *Child & Family Social Work*, 25(1), 173–181.

Kerr, L. & Cossar, J. (2014). Attachment interventions with foster and adoptive parents: A systematic review. *Child Abuse Review (Chichester, England: 1992)*, 23(6), 426–439.

Liu, Q-X., Fang, X-Y., Yan, N., Zhou, Z-K., Yuan, X-J., Lan, J., & Liu, C-Y. (2015). Multi-family group therapy for adolescent Internet addiction: Exploring the underlying mechanisms. *Addictive Behaviors*, 42, 1–8.

Paine, A., Perra, O., Anthony, R., & Shelton, K. (2020). Charting the trajectories of adopted children's emotional and behavioral problems: The impact of early adversity and postadoptive parental warmth. *Development and Psychopathology*, 1–15. https://www.researchgate.net/publication/341151578_Charting_the_trajectories_of_adopted_children%27s_emotional_and_behavioral_problems_The_impact_of_early_adversity_and_postadoptive_parental_warmth.

Pascoe, P., Carlisle, L., Creevy, C., Mackelprang, E., & Rastall, E. (2016). 4.26 Use of multifamily group therapy in long-term inpatient child and adolescent psychiatry program. *Journal of the American Academy of Child and Adolescent Psychiatry*, 55(10), S171.

Perry, B. D. & Dobson C. L. (2012). The neurosequential model of therapeutics. In J. Ford. & C. Courtois. (Eds.), *Treating complex traumatic stress disorder in children and adolescents*. Guilford Press.

Perry, B. D. & Szalavitz, M. (2008). *The boy who was raised as a dog: And other stories from a child psychiatrist's notebook: What traumatized children can teach us about loss, love, and healing*. Basic Books.

Pinto, C. (2019). Looked after and adopted children: Applying the latest science to complex biopsychosocial formulations. *Adoption and Fostering*, 43(3), 294–309. doi:10.1177/0308575919856173.

Reilly, T. & Platz, L. (2004). Post-adoption service needs of families with special needs children: Use, helpfulness, and unmet needs. *Journal of Social Service Research*, 30(4), 51–67.

Riedel Bowers, N. & Bowers, A. (Eds.) (2013). *Play therapy with families, a collaborative approach to healing*. Jason Aronson.

Rowell, K. (2012). *Love me, feed me: The adoptive parents guide to ending the worry of weight, picky eating, power struggles and more*. Family Feeding Dynamics LLC.

Schaefer, C. & Drewes, A. (2013). *The powers of play: Twenty core agents of change*. John Wiley.

Selakovic, M., Galanis, D., Frankiadaki, E., Theodoropoulou, P., & Pomini, V. (2020). T187. Athens multifamily therapy project (A-MFTP) provides systemic multifamily group therapy to youths who have experienced first psychotic episode (FEP) and their families. *Schizophrenia Bulletin*, 46(Suppl 1), S303.

Selwyn, J., Wijedasa, D., & Meakings, S. (2016). *Beyond the Adoption Order: Challenges, interventions and adoption disruption. Research report. University of Bristol School for Policy Studies Hadley Centre for Adoption and Foster Care Studies.* University of Bristol School for Policy Studies Hadley Centre for Adoption and Foster Care Studies. https://assets.publishing.service.gov.uk/gov ernment/uploads/system/uploads/attachment_data/file/301889/Final_Report_-_ 3rd_April_2014v2.pdf.

Steinglass, P., Ostroff, J. S., & Stahl Steinglass, A. (2011). Multiple family groups for adult cancer survivors and their families: A 1-day workshop model. *Family Process*, 50(3), 393–409. www.ncbi.nlm.nih.gov/pmc/articles/PMC4532272/.

Stock, L., Spielhofer, T., & Gieve, M. (2016). *Independent evidence review of post-adoption support interventions: Research report*. The Tavistock Institute of Human Relations (TIHR). Department of Education. http://cdn.basw.co.uk/up load/basw_73202-3.pdf.

Sweeney, D., Baggerly, J., & Dee, R. C. (2014). *Group play therapy: A dynamic approach*. Routledge.

Thorngren, J. M. & Kleist, D. M. (2002). Multiple family group therapy: An inter-personal/postmodern approach. *The Family Journal*, 10(2), 167–176. doi:10.1177/ 1066480702102006.

Webb, S. (2008). Adoption, play therapy and attachment focussed family therapy. *Adoption Today*, October/November, 26–47.

Zarbo, C., Tasca, G. A., Cattafi, F., & Compare, A. (2016). *Integrative psy-chotherapy works*. The National Center for Biotechnology Information. www. ncbi.nlm.nih.gov/pmc/articles/PMC4707273/.

17 Play Therapy Groups with Neurodiverse Children

Cary McAdams Hamilton and Sarah M. Moran

Neurodiversity has increased recognition in the mental health field and research is showing that attuning to and being aware of how to work with neurodiverse populations is necessary (Goodman-Scott & Lambert, 2015). Children diagnosed with Attention Deficit Hyperactivity Disorder (ADHD), Sensory Processing Disorder (SPD), and Autism Spectrum Disorder (ASD) are often participating in mental health treatment due to the myriad of behavioral and emotional challenges present (Hansen et al., 2000). The intersection of play therapy theory and techniques with neurodiverse populations through group play therapy is the focus of this chapter.

Attention Deficit Hyperactivity Disorder

ADHD is one of the most commonly diagnosed disorders in children in the United States, with prevalence rates ranging from 9 to 11% (National Center for Health Statistics & Centers for Disease Control and Prevention [CDC], 2015; Nielsen et al., 2017; Philion, 2019; Robinson et al., 2017; Wexler, 2013). Current research elucidates that ADHD is a developmental disorder which commonly presents with co-occurring anxiety, depression, sensory processing challenges, learning disabilities, developmental coordination challenges, problems with self-regulation, and/or other neurodiverse diagnoses, including autism (Berger et al., 2013; Delgado-Lobete et al., 2020; Dodson, 2016; Lane & Reynolds, 2019; Philion, 2019). This demonstrates the need for treating this population from a play therapy neurodiverse lens. This chapter focuses on the diagnosis of ADHD, which often has an overlap with sensory processing challenges. We are not accounting for autism in this chapter.

The deficits of ADHD highlight dysfunction in multiple areas of daily life, including education, leisure activities, social participation, and engaging in play; this indicates the need for extra support around social engagement, self-regulation, and the individual's ability to successfully communicate their needs (Lane & Reynolds, 2019; Mimouni-Bloch et al., 2018; Nielsen et al., 2017). Parents frequently perceive that their children with ADHD are failing to be successful in public and in peer relationships,

DOI: 10.4324/9781003094531-17

resulting in increased conflict and overly punitive behavior imparted on the child (Leben, 2015). Mimouni-Bloch et al. (2018) articulated what is frequently reflected in the research, that "ADHD can profoundly affect the academic achievements, well-being, and social interactions of children" (p. 69). Due to the impact ADHD has on executive functioning skills including: attention, focus, planning, sequencing, organizing, initiating, emotion regulation, mental flexibility, time management, impulse control, and delaying gratification; the focus for treatment in this population is the development of social skills and self-regulation (Berger et al., 2013; Leben, 2015; Panagiotidi et al., 2018; Philion, 2019). ADHD has long been known to cause significant social-emotional delays and emotional distress of rejection sensitivity in peer groups resulting in low self-esteem, self-doubt, and negative self-concept (Berger et al., 2013; Dodson, 2016; Leben, 2015). It is the complexity of this diagnosis and the effects it has on multiple areas of daily living that factor into the mental health of the child and family.

Sensory Overlap

A conducted literature review preparing for this chapter highlighted the need to address the sensory systems and comorbidity rates associated with a diagnosis of ADHD. Mimouni-Bloch et al. (2018) found that "daily function difficulties in children with ADHD are significantly more common when there are comorbid sensory modulation difficulties" (p. 73). Other researchers implied that understanding the overlap of sensory processing challenges with ADHD is imperative to conceptualizing the comprehensive nature of this condition (Goodman-Scott & Lambert, 2015; Lane & Reynolds, 2019; Panagiotidi et al., 2018). Applying key strategies to address movement, body regulation, and modulation are key components to the group process when working with this population (Nielsen et al., 2017; Vaisvaser, 2019). Therefore, it is important to attune to the developmental delay of sensory sensitivities directly when treating ADHD. Relatedly, Sensory Processing Disorder (SPD) is defined as:

> A neurophysiologic condition in which sensory input either from the environment or from one's body is poorly detected, modulated, or interpreted and/or to which atypical responses are observed. Pioneering occupational therapist and psychologist A. Jean Ayres, Ph.D., likened SPD to a neurological "traffic jam" that prevents certain parts of the brain from receiving the information needed to interpret sensory information correctly.
>
> (STAR Institute, 2020).

It is noteworthy that SPD is a neurodevelopmental disorder that can be independent of ADHD and has significant mental health impacts on anxiety, depression, and mood disorders in children (Goodman-Scott & Lambert, 2015). The research overwhelmingly demonstrates the corollary that the majority of children diagnosed with ADHD have sensory sensitivities that directly impact their ability to meet developmental milestones, compared to those of their peers who are neurotypical (Delgado-Lobete et al., 2020; Lane & Reynolds, 2019; Mimouni-Bloch et al., 2018; Panagiotidi et al., 2018; Sanz-Cervera et al., 2017). As such, it is necessary to address both sensory systems *and* social development in treatment, which can be achieved through group dynamics that facilitate prosocial learning and acquisition of skills necessary for interpersonal functioning.

Multimodal Treatment

In neurodevelopmental disorders, it has been found that multimodal forms of treatment often have the most long-lasting impacts on well-being and social functioning in interpersonal relationships (Dodson, 2016; Philion, 2019). For children with ADHD, other services (beyond mental health treatment) may include occupational therapists (OTs), vision therapy, pediatricians, child psychiatrists, neuropsychologists, school supports/accommodations, and parent/family resources and support (Philion, 2019). Therapeutic group work with ADHD is supported by social learning theory found in group processes (Hansen et al., 2000). Specifically, as individuals with ADHD often have social skills deficits or difficulties with behavioral management, group formats can address these domains by enhancing connection, increasing awareness of self and others, modeling healthy social interactions, and promoting skill development for their future interpersonal relationships. The inherent social dynamics of a group facilitate an experiential process that enables one to problem solve, try out new skills, and receive regulation within peer relationships. Thus, the therapeutic change is that of an internal locus of control focus and not just behavior change (Hansen et al., 2000; Landreth, 2012; Landreth & Sweeney, 2001). Relatedly, one challenge for families with children and loved ones with ADHD is the time and effort required to engage and commit to multimodal treatment(s), including group therapy. Although groups take advanced planning and coordination, the key aspects of group work meet the therapeutic benefits for this population and are therefore clinically indicated and recommended. For children with ADHD, it is often a benefit to engage in concurrent therapeutic strategies, which may include individual counselor and/or services with other providers. It is the multimodal approach that supports sustainability and provides the most beneficial impact for the child's diagnosis and symptom reduction (Dodson, 2016; Philion, 2019).

Social Skill Deficits

Research suggests the social deficits inherent to SPD, combined with the core features of ADHD, can intensify symptoms of anxiety and depression in children and adolescents (Lane & Reynolds, 2019). Given these negative outcomes and the high comorbidity between SPD and ADHD, the complex nature of ADHD and social skills development can be addressed by using the group therapy process (Delgado-Lobete et al., 2020; Mimouni-Bloch et al., 2018; Nielsen et al., 2017; Philion, 2019; Sanz-Cervera et al., 2017).

For elementary school children between the ages of 7–10, social skill development and social-cue learning patterns are acquired through interacting with others, usually in educational or other group settings. Indeed, key features of this developmental state include socialization, peer acceptance, people-pleasing, and finding a sense of belonging (Ray, 2016). Groups with this age range (approximately 7–10 years old) would be most effective for children with comorbid ADHD/SPD, as the research indicates a shift in brain development at the onset of adolescence (Berger et al., 2013; Ray, 2016). There is often a maturational delay for those diagnosed with ADHD of one to three years which impacts social-emotional development (Berger et al., 2013; Wexler, 2013). However, group dynamics will remain pertinent for older children and adolescents diagnosed with ADHD, with adjustments made for size and social relatedness of the group.

In various social contexts, children and adolescents with ADHD may perceive that they "do not fit in" with their peers. Research suggests individuals with ADHD have greater difficulty regulating emotions compared to their neurotypical classmates, which contributes to negative peer interactions and perceived lack of social acceptance (Dodson, 2016; Goodman-Scott & Lambert, 2015; Hansen et al., 2000; Leben, 2015; Philion, 2019). As Dodson (2016) articulated, "children with ADHD hear 20,000 additional critical or corrective messages before their twelfth birthday when compared to neurotypical children" (p. 9). This encourages the need for prosocial groups that focus on improving the ADHD child's ability to meet more of the social expectations of their peer groups.

Play Therapy and ADHD

Play therapy is a developmentally appropriate treatment for children that uses the child's natural language, play (Landreth, 2012). A common approach to working with the ADHD population is to understand each child's neurodevelopmental delays and strengths in the context of play therapy. As such, play therapists with a background in neurodiversity can utilize non-directive and directive approaches in therapeutic work with ADHD.

Therapists should consider working from an integrative perspective, with foundational child-centered play therapy (CCPT) as the therapeutic guidepost. The CCPT group play therapist can provide the opportunity for all, including children with ADHD "to be viewed as a positive and growing self, while also experiencing the evaluation of the other group members within an atmosphere of permissiveness and acceptance" (Landreth & Sweeney, 2001, p. 184). Children with ADHD are highly creative, out-of-the-box thinkers and problem solvers that flourish in the playroom. It is the supportive, regulated, and unconditional positive regard of the therapist that builds up self-esteem and confidence. Of note, it is imperative that the therapist be in a regulated state so that all children, and especially those with neurodevelopmental disorders such as ADHD, SPD, or ASD, can have a sense of safety and security in the playroom. Transferring this practice to group treatment is necessary as the goal of CCPT is to support self-esteem and encourage positive self-concept, particularly within a peer-supported group context.

Robinson et al. (2017) indicates that "CCPT is shown to have effects on behaviors related to both the inattentive and hyperactive/impulsive subtypes of ADHD" (p. 81). Specifically, CCPT has been found to support emotion regulation, communication skills, intrinsic motivation, self-expression, and decision making and problem-solving skills (Landreth, 2012; Landreth & Sweeney, 2001; Swank & Smith-Adcock, 2018). Similarly, using more directive play therapy can support children with ADHD in need of more specific directives such as: playing psychoeducational games, reading therapeutic books, or learning specific emotion regulation skills through role-modeling and repeat exercises. The language of CCPT is notable for its alignment of unconditional positive regard and belief that the child is able to achieve success on their own (Landreth, 2012). It is the combination of directive structure and non-directive language used throughout the group process that establishes the security and sense of felt safety that this integrative model provides all children, and especially those with ADHD.

Group Play Therapy for ADHD

The group play therapy environment "allows children the opportunity to discover that their peers may be struggling too, which helps deconstruct the barriers that children have of feeling alone in their pain" (Landreth & Sweeney, 2001, p. 201). Therapeutic groups are beneficial to the ADHD population as the relational patterns and comradery built around similar challenges promote connectedness and a sense of belonging to individuals that frequently feel isolated and rejected (Dodson, 2016; Leben, 2015; Nielsen et al., 2017). Group work for children and adolescents with ADHD would additionally provide consistency and necessary repetition, which is needed to form new neuronal integration patterns. It is this ongoing development of increasing neural connections through the relational group dynamic that provides the support and encouragement needed for ADHD social development. As Donald Hebb (1949) noted, "neurons that fire together wire together" (as cited in Siegel & Bryson, 2011).

A co-therapy approach with this population allows for several therapeutic factors to be imparted. These include promotion of teamwork, role modeling of appropriate communication and social skills between therapists and within the group dynamics. It is recommended to utilize co-facilitators in group treatment as this provides more opportunity for co-regulation and a tag-team approach to managing inattention and impulsive behaviors characteristic of ADHD (Nielsen et al., 2017; Philion, 2019; Vaisvaser, 2019). The therapeutic goals of group treatment should be focused interventions that target 1) proximal awareness and body regulation, 2) recognition of facial expressions, 3) identification, expression, and effective communication of emotion (verbal and nonverbal), 4) acceptance of others and self, 5) increased confidence and self-esteem, and 6) baseline understanding of expected societal, interpersonal skills.

Integration of Sensory Dynamics

ADHD populations, especially those with a predominantly hyperactive/impulsive presentation, are usually active with frequent body movements and psychomotor agitation. Thus, it is important the therapist has enough room and space to allow for unpredictable moving bodies and materials. Multi-sensory environments can facilitate enhanced communication skills, increased relaxation, increased alertness to task, as well as a reduction in anxiety (Fletcher et al., 2019; Goodman-Scott & Lambert, 2015). To mimic multi-sensory environments, we recommend obtaining materials and items to promote self-regulation as a part of the group process. Relatedly, it is suggested that therapists encourage creativity and promote skill development through modeling of healthy emotion regulation and flexibility, especially given the nature of disinhibition often displayed in ADHD. As such, it is recommended to implement a CCPT-informed group treatment targeting executive functioning and social skills acquisition through the experiential nature of group process, expanding the client's "perceptual awareness of self and others' intentions, conveyed through creative modalities involving sensorimotor experiences" (Vaisvaser, 2019, p. 2).

Depending on the focus of the group, visual props (such as hula hoops or tape on the floor) may be indicated (Vaisvaser, 2019); this can facilitate neurobiological attunement with one's physical space, as well as increase understanding of boundaries with others. Additional items that can be helpful in a variety of group formats include: bean bags, stretchy bands, stress balls, miscellaneous tactile fidgets, sensory bins (rice, beans, sand), weighted vests/lap pads, stability balls/medicine balls, sensory walk items (tape, blocks, mats, balance boards, color pressure boards), swings, rockers, textural furniture, and aromatherapy (Fletcher et al., 2019; Nielsen et al., 2017; Philion, 2019). Thus, the use of sensory-engaging activities promotes further opportunities for integration of the non-neurotypical ADHD brain, particularly through "bottom-up" sensory and relational skill development (Vaisvaser, 2019).

Group Considerations

When looking to form a group it is important to account for some similarities of age, personality, level of regulation, and previous success at group work. Groups should aim for 4 or 6 participants, depending on the skills of the therapists, ADHD subtype, gender, and age of the children (Landreth & Sweeney, 2001). Addressing these factors will ensure a more successful group process. To illustrate, an even number of group participants will increase the possibilities of effective dyadic work and prevent ongoing social isolation within the group dynamic by consistently providing opportunities for peer engagement.

Consideration for length of session and number of sessions is limited by the developmental age range, space/location to be used, and what works for the families. In general, sessions can range from 60–90 minutes, weekly, for 10–12 weeks; the therapist must note that it takes time for the group dynamics to coalesce, which is necessary for this population's success. Given the delayed maturation of social-emotional development in individuals with ADHD (Berger et al., 2013; Wexler, 2013), the use of novelty in directives and repetition of concepts within the group setting is clinically indicated (Leben, 2015). Breaking down the tasks of skill-based learning into smaller steps is helpful for this population to sustain attention and practice patience (Leben, 2015). The promotion and generalization of group work skills to families' needs highlights the benefit of working alongside other individuals facing the same challenges, as humans do better with mimicking and role-modeling than in individual approaches. The social dynamic of group work is particularly relevant to this population, and can accelerate skills acquisition, due to the development of successful peer relationships in the group microcosm. To further this skill development, families should be encouraged to meet outside of the therapeutic group to share resources and a felt sense of belonging (Landreth & Sweeney, 2001).

As forementioned, the ADHD population has received more negative input from others about their behaviors than neurotypical children, which invariably contributes to their negative self-concept and low self-esteem (Dodson, 2016; Goodman-Scott & Lambert, 2015; Hansen et al., 2000; Leben, 2015). As such, the language used within the group requires that the therapists are aware of the shame-related concepts in societal statements and will actively work to not use these in the group dynamic. Therapists must have awareness that behaviors will often come from the need for sensory outlets; they must be flexible with some allowance for the behavior and redirection, if needed, to maintain a safe environment. This most often is observed, recognized, and modeled by the therapist using self to ensure safety of the group. Vaisvaser (2019) provided this example "You are here with us, you want to be seen, we see you, but this is not allowed" (p. 4) to be a reflective, inclusive, and prosocial redirection of the child's behavior. This is consistent with the notion that co-therapists practice from a CCPT lens that is relationally focused.

Establishment of group rules follow the basic steps of structure, routine, and expectations of other group settings. It is important to pre-establish some safety and boundary rules for groups and allow opportunities for children to develop their own group rules. This provides participants some ownership and peer alignment to follow in the group process.

Creation of an initiated start and end routine engages attention and promotes containment of the group process (Hansen et al., 2000; Leben, 2015; Vaisvaser, 2019). Group engagement should then be followed by a sensorimotor activity for regulation, such as: a sensory walk, hula hooping, exercise bands, yoga, animal walks, or cross body throwing/rolling activities (use of weighted or feather-light items). The therapist can engage the group to do 1–2 of these activities, as a group or in dyads, while identifying (through the use of reflection) each child/dyad's progress and actions. The therapists can then transition the group to applying more executive function skills through psychoeducation or bibliotherapy while participants have access to the available sensory manipulatives. Reading aloud to children of all ages can improve listening skills and support relational bonds (Landreth, 2012; Philion, 2019). To promote integration of sensory experiences and executive functioning skills learned, we suggest pairing two activities together. Other activities can include art expression on vertical surfaces or oversized paper to promote right-left brain integration, creativity, and expression. Art expression or body regulation activities can be done while listening to music or singing a song as a group (Vaisvaser, 2019). Having the group create rhythmic melodic songs about the skills they are learning can help reinforce learning and increase success outside of the group. Lastly, each session will close with a predetermined ritual directed by the therapists (Leben, 2015; Vaisvaser, 2019). The predictability, consistency, and structure of this group formula will ensure a felt sense of safety and implement body-before-brain regulation that is crucial for meeting the needs of neurodiverse children (Hansen et al., 2000). The use of CCPT with this population in particular encourages an internalized sense of achievement and development of self-control, instead of the typical focus on externalized behaviors, thus creating greater and longer lasting change (Hansen et al., 2000; Landreth & Sweeney, 2001).

Case Study

This case study examines how to build rapport, establish group norms and healthy boundaries when beginning group play therapy with neurodiverse children who have been diagnosed with ADHD. A group of six children diagnosed with ADHD between the ages of 6–8 years old presented for group play therapy with two co-therapists, both of whom specialized in working with neurodiversity and sensory processing challenges. The parents of the children had reported issues such as disruptive behavior at school, missed homework assignments, forgetfulness, roughhousing with siblings at home, and climbing on furniture. They reported ongoing academic and peer challenges.

During the first group session, participants worked to develop rapport and to create shared group rules for confidentiality, respect, and inclusion. During this group conversation children were seated on wiggle seats to allow for adherence to staying in a circle, engaging their vestibular, proprioceptive, and tactile senses for improved focus and listening. Clinicians then introduced a directive activity of a tape maze to facilitate mindfulness/focus through specific sensory activity. For this group, to engage the most movement and practice, each individual child moved through a tape maze on the floor with a variety of additional tasks to complete, repeating the exercise with increased success. Clinicians worked with each child on motivation or not using negative self-talk, reflecting instead on the progress being made and encouragement to push through. If a child struggled, one clinician engaged the child with encouragement and one-on-one connection both verbally and physically with presence. The other clinician fostered the other children to manage space, body, and actions, encouraging the positive dialogue between the children as they completed the exercise. The group then transitioned to free play with sensory toys/materials for 15 minutes, with each therapist taking time to reflect each child's processing and facilitation of social interactions between group participants using CCPT language.

Clinicians then directed the group to select one tactile play material (kinetic sand, model magic, sands alive, or playdoh) to manipulate while the clinicians provided bibliotherapy on the specific topic of growth mindset/flexible thinking. One therapist read out loud, while the other therapist moved between members, giving eye contact, smiling, encouraging listening and use of sensory material, and navigating any child's need for more sensory input. The session closed with a group discussion of the concepts of flexible thinking, while modeling developmentally appropriate social skills, and interpersonal boundaries. Each child was given the opportunity to reflect an idea or concept learned and how they will apply this outside of the group. The group was then led out of session using animal walks to waiting parents.

Conclusion

Although there exists significant research on neurodiversity and its impact on social functioning for ADHD and SPD, there is little about group dynamic work. The aim of implementing sensory tools and materials into group play therapy for children with ADHD and sensory processing challenges is consistent with goals often outlined in Occupational Therapy for neurodiverse children (Delgado-Lobete et al., 2020; Lane & Reynolds, 2019; Philion, 2019; Vaisvaser, 2019). The addition of a co-facilitated CCPT group for children with ADHD approximately 7–10 years old serves to enhance skill-development and establish a much-needed sense of belonging and acceptance for children who otherwise feel ostracized or different from their neurotypical peers. The relational dynamics of group therapy facilitate neuro-integration (via flexible and co-regulated state in the group process) allows the "ADHD brain" to successfully develop healthier social skills, improve interpersonal relationships, and increase self-regulation.

References

Berger, I., Slobodin, O., Aboud, M., Melamed, J., & Cassuto, H. (2013, October). Maturational delay in ADHD: Evidence from CPT. *Frontiers in Human Neuroscience*, 7(69), 1–11. doi:10.3389/fnhum.2013.00691.

Delgado-Lobete, L., Pértega-Díaz, S., Santos-del-Riego, S., & Montes-Montes, R. (2020). Sensory processing patterns in developmental coordination disorder, attention deficit hyperactivity disorder and typical development. *Research in Developmental Disabilities*, 100. doi:10.1016/j.ridd.2020.103608.

Dodson, W. W. (2016). Emotional regulation and rejection sensitivity. *Attention*, 8–11.

Fletcher, T., Anderson-Seidens, J., Wagner, H., Linyard, M., & Nicolette, E. (2019). Caregivers' perceptions of barriers and supports for children with sensory processing disorders. *Australian Occupational Therapy Journal*, 66, 617–626. doi:10.1111/1440-1630.12601.

Goodman-Scott, E. & Lambert, S. F. (2015). Professional counseling for children with sensory processing disorder. *The Professional Counselor*, 5(2), 273–292.

Hansen, S., Meissler, K., & Ovens, R. (2000). Kids together: A group play therapy model for children with ADHD symptomatology. *Journal of Child and Adolescent Group Therapy*, 10(4), 191–211.

Landreth, G. L. (2012). *The art of the relationship* (3rd ed.). Brunner & Routledge.

Landreth, G. L. & Sweeney, D. S. (2001). Child-centered group play therapy. In G. L. Landreth (Ed.), *Innovations in play therapy: Issues, process, and social populations* (pp. 181–202). Brunner & Routledge.

Lane, S. J. & Reynolds, S. (2019). Sensory over-responsivity as an added dimension in ADHD. *Frontiers in Integrative Neuroscience*, 13(40). doi:10.3389/fnint.2019.00040

Leben, N. (2015). Directive group play therapy for children with attention-deficit/hyperactivity disorder. In H. G. Kaduson & C. E. Schaefer (Eds.), *Short term play therapy for children* (3rd ed., pp. 325–352). Guilford Press.

Mimouni-Bloch, A., Offek, H., Rosenblum, S., Posener, I., Silman, Z., & Engel-Yeger, B. (2018). Association between sensory modulation and daily activity function of children with attention deficit/hyperactivity disorder and children with typical development. *Research in Developmental Disabilities*, 83, 69–76. doi:10.1016/j.ridd.2018.08.002.

National Center for Health Statistics & Centers for Disease Control and Prevention. (2015). *Data and statistics about ADHD.* Centers for Disease Control and Prevention. www.cdc.gov/ncbddd/adhd/data.html.

Nielsen, S. K., Kelsch, K., & Miller, K. (2017). Occupational therapy interventions for children with attention deficit hyperactivity disorder: A systematic review. *Occupational Therapy In Mental Health*, 33(1), 70–80. doi:10.1080/0164212X.2016.1211060.

Panagiotidi, M., Overton, P. G., & Stafford, T. (2018). The relationship between ADHD traits and sensory sensitivity in the general population. *Comprehensive Psychology*, 80, 179–185. doi:10.1016/j.comppsych.2017.10.008.

Philion, D. (2019, March). Comprehensive treatment for children with attention deficit/hyperactivity disorder. *Play Therapy Magazine*, 14(1), 10–14.

Ray, D. C. (Ed.) (2016). *A therapist's guide to child development: The extraordinarily normal years.* Routledge/Taylor & Francis Group.

Robinson, A., Simpson, C., & Hott, B. L. (2017). The effects of child-centered play therapy on the behavioral performance of three first grade students with ADHD. *International Journal of Play Therapy*, 26(2), 73–83. doi:10.1037/pla0000047.

Sanz-Cervera, P., Pastor-Cerezuela, G., González-Sala, F., Tárraga-Minguez, R., & Fernández Andrés, M.-I. (2017). Sensory processing in children with autism spectrum disorder and/or attention deficit hyperactivity disorder in the home and classroom contexts. *Frontiers in Psychology*, 8(1772). doi:10.3389/fpsyg.2017.01772

Siegel, D. J. & Bryson, T. P. (2011). *The whole-brain child: 12 revolutionary strategies to nurture your child's developing mind.* Random House.

STAR Institute. (2020). *What is Sensory Processing Disorder?* SPDStar. www.spdstar.org/basic/understanding-sensory-processing-disorder.

Swank, J. M. & Smith-Adcock, S. (2018, October). On-task behavior with children with attention deficit hyperactivity disorder: Examining treatment effectiveness of play therapy interventions. *International Journal of Play Therapy*, 27(4), 187–197.

Vaisvaser, S. (2019, March). Moving along and beyond the spectrum: Creative group therapy for children with autism. *Frontiers in Psychology*, 10(417). doi:10.3389/fpsyg.2019.00417

Wexler, B. E. (2013, July–September). Integrated brain and body exercises for ADHD and related problems with attention and executive function. *International Journal of Gaming and Computer-Mediated Simulations*, 3(3), 10–26. doi:10.4018/jgcms.2013070102.

18 Play Therapy Group Supervision

Jennifer Taylor

Mental health professionals are well-versed in the benefits of supervision while they are developing new skills and/or dealing with challenging cases throughout their psychotherapy careers. Supervision is one component of clinical competency and is typically required as part of graduate degree programs and specialized postgraduate training programs. Statements about obtaining adequate supervision are included in the Code of Ethics for the American Counseling Association (2014), the National Association for Social Workers (2017), and the American Psychological Association (2017).

In play therapy, clinicians often refer to the Association for Play Therapy (APT) for the education, direct practice, and supervision requirements for credentialing as a Registered Play Therapist (2019). However, professionals who are not pursuing credentialing as a Registered Play Therapist are still ethically required by their professional code of ethics to obtain appropriate training and supervision. For those clinicians adhering to APT's (2019) guidelines for the Registered Play Therapist credential one of the supervision specific requirements (as of this writing) includes thirty-five hours of in-person or distance supervision received from a Registered Play Therapist-Supervisor (a person who has additional training and experience providing play therapy services). Ten of those thirty-five hours may be obtained in a group format and it is those hours of group supervision that are the focus of this chapter.

In this chapter, the reasons that clinicians seek out group supervision as well as the benefits to their clinical practice are explored. A range of methods provide examples of how supervisors can facilitate group play therapy supervision sessions. Several theoretical components are summarized to provide a foundation for how to conceptualize play therapy cases with group members who have different levels of experience and professional training. These concepts are then demonstrated through a case example from a group supervision session so they can be applied to play therapy practice. Together, these methods form a latticework of theory that provide both structure and flexibility for group play therapy supervision.

DOI: 10.4324/9781003094531-18

Overview of Group Supervision

Supervision is explained as "the relationship between supervisor and supervisee in which the responsibility and accountability for the development of competence, demeanor and ethical practice take place" (National Association for Social Workers & Association of Social Work Boards, 2013, p. 6). Group supervision, by extension, includes dyads, triads, or larger peer groups with a variety of structures. In group supervision, participants benefit from the collective wisdom of each of the group members, with the supervisor remaining responsible for upholding competent and ethical practices for all involved.

There are many reasons why clinicians seek out group supervision experiences, but the most frequently cited is the desire to hear additional cases, experiences, and feedback from more than one person (Borders, 2012). Successful supervision groups have characteristics such as trust, caring and acceptance, a sense of belonging, and being valued (Davis et al., 2018). As a result, many clinicians participate in groups for more hours than required by their boards because the groups meet their goals for building community and solving challenging cases (Borders, 2012). Play therapy supervisees reported the highest satisfaction levels based on their supervisors' years of experience and strong professional identity as a play therapist (VanderGast & Hinkle, 2015). Group supervision was not specifically noted, but it is plausible that play therapy supervision groups help develop a sense of professional identity.

While satisfaction with group supervision is important, the efficacy of the process is paramount. Group supervision has been shown to be as effective as individual supervision in learning clinical skills (Lanning, 1971), empathetic responding (Averitte, 1989), and equal to combined group and individual supervision (Ray & Altekruse, 2000). A notable limitation in play therapy supervision research is the reliance on surveys or qualitative studies, research that only involved pre-graduate level students, or examined specific interventions, and a lack of a comprehensive look at the effectiveness of postgraduate play therapy supervision or long-term effectiveness (Donald et al., 2015). Other research examining group supervision has demonstrated efficacy. In a study of web-based supervision with school counselors, counselor self-esteem and case conceptualization skills were both increased following twelve online group supervision sessions (Butler & Constantine, 2006). In Turkey, structured peer group supervision was shown to increase counseling skills of focusing, empathy, reflection of contents and feelings, asking questions, and confrontation (Atik & Erkan Atik, 2019). A structured peer group supervision of pre-doctoral psychology students examined group supervision and found that it mirrored the benefits of group psychotherapy including interpersonal learning, universality, imitative behavior, and imparting information. The additional benefits for the counseling profession included self-care practices, self-reflective practices, integrating theoretical perspectives, and case conceptualization skills (Schumann et al., 2020).

It is clear that clinicians enjoy group supervision and that it is effective for professional development, but supervisors also need examples of how to facilitate group supervision. The Center for Play Therapy at the University of North Texas employs a "doing and observing" model of learning child-centered play therapy supervision in which therapists have sessions with child clients, watch other therapists sessions through a two-way mirror, and then discuss all of the cases in a small group format (Bratton et al., 1993, p. 72). This format of group supervision, in place since 1992, reports benefits that include peer feedback, sharing of creative ideas, increased self-awareness, and encouraged peer-to-peer supervision skills (Bratton et al., 1993). Allen, Folger, and Pehrsson (2007) described the development of child-centered play therapy skills as a three-step model with the initial focus on learning the skill of tracking, then on reflecting feelings and objects, and finally reflecting the clients' own feelings. A similar method of doing and observing is done through role-play with graduate level students learning the Oaklander method of play therapy. In this method, students work in dyads or triads to role-play therapists, clients, and observers, and practice play therapy interventions using picture cards, drawing, clay, sand tray, and puppets. Group members reported that these experiences were substantially helpful in providing, "awareness, insights, and tools" for their play therapy practice (Mortola, 2019, p. 73).

Outside of the university setting, supervision groups offer opportunities for discussion of cases and for experiential play or expressive arts-based interventions that may enhance the skills and experience of the group. The use of metaphors in supervision has been identified as helpful in the supervision process to facilitate case conceptualization skills (Guiffrida et al., 2007). Guiffrida et al. furthered that metaphoric activities in supervision may allow supervisors and supervisees to develop a shared language, facilitate deeper understandings of relationships, encourage supervisees to find their own solutions to cases, and also share more challenging cases in less time (p. 398). LEGO® Serious Play® (LSP) has been used with supervisees by offering a directive prompt, building a metaphoric model out of bricks, telling a story about it, and then discussing and reflecting on its applications to their cases (Peabody, 2015).

The sand tray offers an additional opportunity for the exploration of symbols and metaphors in supervision groups. Sandtray directives are "easily modified to be respectful of and responsive to the supervisee's developmental level" (Perryman et al., 2016, p. 186). One potential prompt is to build a world in the sand focused on a specific client situation and then process it from different points of view. Another option is through the use of a directive prompt where the entire supervision group co-creates one sand tray together (Hartwig & Bennett, 2017). Directive prompts can also be useful to address specific concerns within a group.

A music-inspired poetic sharing technique was employed in a supervision group experiencing conflict among participants (Davis et al., 2018). In that example, each group member wrote down words/phrases that came to mind while they listened to a piece of instrumental music together. The group members exchanged lists and then they each created a poem based on the words from the list. After reading each poem aloud to each other, the group reported an increased sense of group cohesion and ability to work together. Additional examples of directive interventions labeled as a "potpourri of playful techniques" as well as guidelines for their selection are included in the book *Supervision Can be Playful* (Drewes & Mullen, 2008, pp. 271–308).

Research and/or Theory on Group Work with Supervision

Supervisors must rely on a theoretical foundation to further navigate the provision of group supervision. Charlie Munger's "latticework of theory" is helpful here to organize the many available theoretical models that describe the process of facilitating group play therapy supervision. Latticework of theory is defined as the "assembling of many big models from many interrelated disciplines into an interrelated structure that resembles a lattice to make better decisions" (Griffin, 2015, p. 190). This philosophy is credited to Charlie Munger, who is a successful investor and business partner to Warren Buffet and not a psychotherapist. And yet, the concept applies well as a way to organize the interrelated concepts at work in group supervision. For example, one latticework of theory is made by assembling together the Integrated Developmental Model, prescriptive play therapy theory, and the Play Therapy Dimensions Model. This is achieved in group supervision when the supervisor prompts one member to pose an initial question or case example and then invites other group members to provide resources or feedback regarding the case conceptualizations. The supervisor may offer additional insights or theoretical perspectives, summarize the options provided and facilitate additional conversations about the nuances in treatment planning for each group member based on the supervisors awareness of each members cases and experience.

One of the more frequently cited supervision models is the Integrated Developmental Model (IDM) which divides clinical development into phases with broad labels of 1) beginning students, 2) intermediate counselors, 3) counselors with two–three years of experience, and then the developers added a fourth category labeled 3i, to represent integration (Stoltenberg & McNeill, 2010). The IDM explains the differences in supervisee needs over the phases where beginning therapists are more dependent on the supervisor and this dependency decreases over time. Ray's (2011) theory on therapist development in child-centered play therapy layers well with the phases of the IDM. This path describes how a therapist initially focuses on learning new skills with expectations of specific directions from the supervisor, then explores interventions or beliefs from other theories or without consulting with the supervisor first, then openly explores Child-centered Play Therapy in comparison to other models, and finally develops a relationship that is more consultative in nature. Stoltenberg and McNeill (2010) note that the phases in the IDM do have limitations and that "this broad view of general developmental skills is too simplistic and does not reflect reality" (p. 22). The authors continue this explanation by citing nuances within the model that explain how a clinician may be at Level 3 in one practice area (depression in adult females), but Level 1 in another (childhood sexual abuse). These variations are clearly evident in play therapy supervision groups where clinicians present with an array of experience in their overall counseling skills as well as their play therapy specific experience. For this reason, the IDM (along with play therapy specific knowledge of therapist development) serve as a starting point for supervisory assessment of clinical skills in a group setting.

Clinicians come to supervision groups from different developmental levels, but also to play therapy groups with a variety of play therapy theoretical orientations. For this reason, a supervisor may include prescriptive play therapy in their latticework of theories. Prescriptive play therapy, as coined by Charles Schaefer, "describes a theoretical approach to play therapy that draws from a variety of modalities and approaches within play therapy in an integrated manner to develop a comprehensive assessment and treatment plan" (Beckley-Forest & Monaco, 2020, p. 4; Kaduson et al., 2020; O'Connor & Schaefer, 2016). Prescriptive play therapy addresses concerns that play therapists may have been exposed to only one or two theoretical models of play therapy in graduate school, but affirms that by having more theoretical options, the therapist is "able to treat a more diverse clientele that matches individual needs to evidence-based practice" (Peabody & Schaeffer, 2016, p. 199). This is different from using all theories at one time. It is the careful selection of the right theory and interventions tailored to each individual client. In the process of group play therapy supervision, a skilled supervisor who has experience using a prescriptive play therapy approach will be able to help less experienced therapists apply that same thought process to their own cases.

The third element in this latticework of theory is the Play Therapy Dimensions Model (PTDM) which provides the structure needed for case conceptualization and treatment planning along with the flexibility of applying different theoretical approaches among supervisees in a group. Supervisors will find within this model a method for the conceptualization of cases on two spectrums – degree of consciousness and degree of directiveness. The two spectrums intersect to form four quadrants: 1) active utilization, 2) open discussion and exploration, 3) non-intrusive responding, and 4) co-facilitation (Gardner & Yasenik, 2012). The quadrants, "provide a window for looking at the possibility of using many play therapy models during one session or across sessions" as well as working from one or all of the four quadrants within one session or over the course of treatment (Gardner & Yasenik, 2008, p. 45). The Play Therapy Dimensions Model works well in a group supervision setting because each member of the group can provide insight based on their own authentic experiences and are not limited by the need to share a common theoretical framework or even level of expertise, but they are grounded in a common desire to meet the needs of the child. The supervisor and all group members come prepared to be fully engaged in the process of evaluating play sessions on this spectrum.

Group Example/Intervention

A distance play therapy supervision group consisting of four members from different states met for one-hour twice per month for approximately one year. The format included time for each clinician to present a case, opportunities for each member to provide insights or feedback to each other with additional insight from the supervisor, and a final review of the case conceptualization.

A composite example of one discussion presented during a group supervision session along with a summary of group member and supervisory input shows how the latticework of theory (Integrated Development Model [IDM], prescriptive play therapy, and Play Therapy Dimensions Model) work together so that each group member has feedback on their individual case, but also learns ways to approach other cases in the future.

Preparation

The supervisor prepares for the session by completing an internal review of the developmental stage of each group member using the IDM. Members included a recent college graduate working in a non-profit agency feeling overwhelmed with complex cases, a clinician experienced with adults but new to play therapy work, a school-based social worker well versed in interventions but feeling less comfortable with theory, and a clinician in private practice well versed in child-centered play therapy but lacking knowledge in directive interventions. In thinking about group members in the context of the IDM, the supervisor knows that the group has one beginning therapist (early Level 2) who may still need a lot of support from the supervisor, one that is at Level 3 working with adults, but Level 1 with children, who is likely to need practical ways to integrate play therapy theories to a well-developed knowledge base, one that is at Level 2 and may be likely to test new techniques without oversight, and one that is a Level 3 and is most likely looking for interesting conversation about case complexities.

Case Presentation

The recent college graduate presents the case of an elementary age child that only wants to play games every session. The child has attended an intake session with his mother and three follow-up individual non-directive play therapy sessions. During these sessions, the child gravitates towards either board games or card games, but cannot tolerate losing. The therapist reports that if the child suffers any setbacks or obstacles during the game, the child manipulates or changes the rules (i.e., "cheats") in order to win. The therapist feels frustrated with the repetitiveness of the sessions and is unsure if she is "doing the right thing" by letting the child win all the time. The therapist had engaged in a basic course on child-centered play therapy in graduate school, has been working in the field for less than a year, and has no trained play therapists as co-workers. The question posed to the group is if non-directive play therapy is recommended in this situation or if a more directive approach would be more effective.

Group Discussion

Each group member has an opportunity to offer their unique perspective and possible applications of different play therapy theories using a prescriptive approach. The experienced therapist (new to play therapy) admits that this has not happened in any sessions thus far, but is curious about the family system and prompts some discussion about the environment that the child is coming from, the personalities of the parents, and ways to incorporate the family into the sessions. The school-based therapist has encountered this problem often and shares the challenges of meeting the expectations from teachers and administrators specific to addressing cheating and school code of conduct. She offers a book suggestion and shares an experience using a directive intervention with puppets to role-play social skills in games. The child-centered therapist offers a theoretical perspective explaining why this behavior would not be considered "cheating" at all and is acceptable in her practice as a way for a child to experience feeling powerful. She is also curious about the child's relationships at home and school and wonders what this behavior might say about the way this child experiences the world.

The presenting therapist offers additional information that the child's mother is loving, but also has high expectations for compliance with rules. She reports that the child doesn't follow directions well and tests her limits by yelling, arguing, or simply ignoring rules. The school has not reported any issues with cheating, but the child struggles with social relationships, doesn't have any close friends, and has low, but passing, grades.

Case Conceptualization and Treatment Planning

Using the Play Therapy Dimensions Model, the supervisor summarizes the questions and suggestions offered (child-centered, filial and family systems, directive, CBT, possibly Gestalt play therapy theories) and rather than recommending one preferred course of treatment, directs a conversation about many possible approaches to the case based on the consciousness and directiveness dimensions of the PTDM. At this point, the child's level of consciousness regarding the "cheating" behavior appears low. The therapists infer that the child may feel powerless at home and inadequate and lonely at school. The group discusses the ways in which tracking statements during sessions address the consciousness dimension with a focus merely on content "you're winning every time" and progress over time to bring more specific awareness to the behavior by saying, "you're enjoying being the winner, you feel powerful". This leads to a discussion of the directiveness dimension and rationale for using a more or less directive approach with this child. This includes continuing a non-directive approach that freely allows the child to change the rules of the game and discussions about how interventions may become more directive as the child's ability to talk about his feelings and environment develop. The discussion continues addressing potential concerns from parents and school staff about cheating and the framing of the behavior as appropriate only "in-session". The supervisor ends with a personal case example involving "cheating" behavior showing the trajectory over many sessions beginning with a child-centered/non-directive approach with content-based tracking. In this case, the child abandoned the cheating behavior voluntarily after a few sessions. With time, the child became receptive to directive social skills interventions and family sessions where additional relationship dynamics could be addressed more openly. This example showcases the flexibility of treatment approaches from a prescriptive play therapy perspective.

Review

After these discussions, the presenting therapist expresses an increased sense of confidence with trusting a non-directive process and explaining the treatment plan to the parent. The adult therapist expressed interest in additional training focused on including family members in play sessions. The school-based therapist expressed an increased openness to the idea of allowing "cheating" in sessions along with specific structuring that the therapy environment had special rules that didn't apply in the classroom. The child-centered play therapist affirmed her belief in this theory, felt renewed in the belief of the therapeutic powers of play, and also explored adding the book that was recommended to her for her waiting room.

In follow-up sessions, the supervisor would revisit the case example to give each member an opportunity to discuss their implementation and practice of the skills and interventions discussed. Also, discussions would consider how changes in the child's level of consciousness might prompt an alternative approach that was more/less directive in nature.

Conclusion

The topic of supervision covers a broad scope of research regarding methodology, theoretical orientations, and specific interventions that are all integral to the process. Supervision has been deemed an effective and widely accepted method for acquiring skills and competencies in the counseling field. The benefits of group supervision include the development of a trusted network of play therapy professionals and the ability to hear and learn from multiple perspectives in a short period of time. This collective wisdom allows supervisees to practice case conceptualization skills and improve treatment planning while simultaneously strengthening their theoretical knowledge base.

In this chapter, the synthesis of different supervision models, interventions, and theories create a latticework of theory as they apply to group play therapy supervision that can be summarized with the metaphor of a lattice-topped apple pie. In group supervision, the supervisor is the crust. The supervisor creates a container for the experience that is grounded in ethical and competent play therapy practice. The group members are all complementary types of apples – similar in that they are all mental health professionals but slightly different in their training, experience, and interests. Three lattice strips represent the Integrated Developmental Model showing the levels of therapist experience (novice, intermediate, and experienced). Four strips that cross in a T-shape form the Play Therapy Dimensions Model representing the continuums of consciousness and directiveness in play therapy modalities. And finally, prescriptive play therapy is represented by smaller strips that are specific to each participant's individual attributes including their competence and wisdom in specialized areas (relational neuroscience, trauma, family systems, etc.). During any group play therapy experience as cases are presented, each participant adds figurative strips to the lattice work. At the end, each person takes an individualized slice of that pie that allows them to take an authentic approach to their play therapy cases based on their level of experience, theoretical orientation, and interests. Each participant might walk away with a slightly different conceptualization of their cases, but each one will be formulated through a prescriptive approach based on the worldly wisdom of a combined group of professionals.

References

Allen, V. B., Folger, W. A., & Pehrsson, D. E. (2007). Reflective process in play therapy: A practical model for supervising counseling students. *Education*, 127, 472–479.

American Counseling Association. (2014). *ACA Code of Ethics*. [PDF File]. Author. www.counseling.org/Resources/aca-code-of-ethics.pdf.

American Psychological Association. (2017). *Ethical Principles of Psychologists and Code of Conduct*. Author. www.apa.org/ethics/code.

Association for Play Therapy. (2019). *Credentialing Standards for the Registered Play Therapist.*™ [PDF File]. Author. https://cdn.ymaws.com/www.a4pt.org/resource/resmgr/credentials/2020_credentials/rpt_standards.pdf.

Atik, G. & Erkan Atik, Z. (2019). Undergraduate counseling trainees' perceptions and experiences related to structured peer group supervision: A mixed method study. *Eurasian Journal of Educational Research*, 82, 101–120.

Averitte, J. (1989). Individual versus group supervision of counselor trainers. (Doctoral dissertation, University of Tennessee, 1988). *Dissertation Abstracts International*, 50, 624.

Beckley-Forest, A. & Monaco, A. (Eds.) (2020). *EMDR with children in the play therapy room: An integrated approach*. Springer.

Borders, L. D. (2012). Dyadic, triadic, and group models of peer supervision/consultation: What are their components, and is there evidence of their effectiveness? *Clinical Psychologist*, 16(2), 59–71. doi:10.1111/j.1742-9552.2012.00046.x

Bratton, S., Landreth, G., & Homeyer, L. (1993). An intensive three day play therapy supervision/training model. *International Journal of Play Therapy*, 2(2), 61–79. doi:10.1037/h0089366

Butler, S. K. & Constantine, M. G. (2006). Web-based peer supervision, collective self-esteem, and case conceptualization ability in school counselor trainees. *Professional School Counseling*, 10(2), 146.

Davis, K. M., Snyder, M. A., & Hartig, N. (2018). Intermodal expressive arts in group supervision. *Journal of Creativity in Mental Health*, 13(1), 68–75. doi:10.1080/15401383.2017.1328294

Donald, E. J., Culbreth, J. R., & Carter, A. W. (2015). Play therapy supervision: A review of the literature. *International Journal of Play Therapy*, 24(2), 59–77. doi:10.1037/a0039104

Drewes, A. A. & Mullen, J. A. (Eds.) (2008). *Supervision can be playful: Techniques for child and play therapist supervisors*. Jason Aronson.

Gardner, K. & Yasenik, L. (2008) When approaches collide: A decision-making model for play therapists. In Drewes, A. A. & Mullen, J. A. (Eds.), *Supervision can be playful: Techniques for child and play therapist supervisors*. Jason Aronson.

Gardner, K. & Yasenik, L. (2012) *Play therapy dimension model: A decision making guide for integrative play therapists*. Jessica Kingsley.

Griffin, Tren. (2015). *Charlie Munger: The complete investor*. Columbia Business School Publishing.

Guiffrida, D. A., Jordan, R., Saiz, S., & Barnes, K. L. (2007). The use of metaphor in clinical supervision. *Journal of Counseling & Development*, 85(4), 393–400. doi:10.1002/j.1556-6678.2007.tb00607.x

Hartwig, E. K. & Bennett, M. M. (2017). Four approaches to using sandtray in play therapy supervision. *International Journal of Play Therapy*, 26(4), 230–238. doi:10.1037/pla0000050

Kaduson, H. G., Cangelosi, D., & Schaeffer, C. E. (Eds.) (2020). *Prescriptive play therapy: Tailoring interventions for specific children*. Guilford Press.

Lanning, W. L. (1971). A study of the relation between group and individual counseling supervision and three relationship measures. *Journal of Counseling Psychology*, 18, 401–406. doi:10.1037/h0031521

Mortola, P. (2019). Play becomes real for adults: Measuring effectiveness of expressive arts media for therapists in training using the Oaklander approach. *Gestalt Review*, 23(1), 67. doi:10.5325/gestaltreview.23.1.0067

National Association of Social Workers. (2017). *Code of Ethics.* Washington, DC: Author. www.socialworkers.org/About/Ethics/Code-of-Ethics/Code-of-Ethics-English.

National Association of Social Workers & Association of Social Work Boards. (2013). *Best Practice Standards in Social Work Supervision.* [PDF File]. Washington, DC: Authors. www.socialworkers.org/LinkClick.aspx?fileticket=GBrLbl4BuwI%3D&portalid=0.

O'Connor, K. J. & Schaefer, C. E. (2016). *Handbook of play therapy.* Wiley & Sons, Inc.

Peabody, M. A. (2015). Building with purpose: Using LEGO SERIOUS PLAY in play therapy supervision. *International Journal of Play Therapy*, 24(1), 30–40. doi:10.1037/a0038607

Peabody, M. A. & Schaefer, C. E. (2016). Towards semantic clarity in play therapy. *International Journal of Play Therapy*, 25(4), 197–202. doi:10.1037/pla0000025

Perryman, K. L., Moss, R. C., & Anderson, L. (2016). Sandtray supervision: An integrated model for play therapy supervision. *International Journal of Play Therapy*, 25(4), 186–196. https://doi.org/10.1037/pla0040288

Ray, D. (2011). Supervision of play therapy. In D. Ray (Ed.), *Advanced play therapy: Essential conditions, knowledge, and skills for child practice* (pp. 243–256). Routledge.

Ray, D. & Altekruse, M. (2000). Effectiveness of group supervision versus combined group and individual supervision. *Counselor Education & Supervision*, 40(1), 19–30. doi:10.1002/j.1556-6978.2000.tb01796.x

Schumann, N. R., Farmer, N. M., Shreve, M. M., & Corley, A. M. (2020). Structured peer group supervision: A safe space to grow. *Journal of Psychotherapy Integration*, 30(1), 108–114.

Stoltenberg, C. D. & McNeill, B. W. (2010). *IDM supervision: An integrative developmental model for supervising counselors and therapists* (3rd ed.). Routledge.

VanderGast, T. S. & Hinkle, M. S. (2015). So happy together? Predictors of satisfaction with supervision for play therapist supervisees. *International Journal of Play Therapy*, 24(2), 92–102. \t "_blank" https://doi.org/10.1037/a0039105

Conclusion

Jessica Stone

Implementing Play Therapy with Groups provides play therapists with information, perspectives, approaches, and ideas regarding the use of play therapy within a group setting. Group play therapy practice models are presented along with a variety of clinical settings and special populations to provide the reader with a host of options to utilize and incorporate into their play therapy repertoire.

This book was initially conceptualized prior to the COVID-19 global pandemic. One of the significant realizations for many during the pandemic was that numerous modalities of play therapy, and in turn group play therapy, are applicable for telehealth as well as in-person groups. Mental health needs have been exacerbated, recognized, and addressed in ways never seen before on such a global level. It is the editors' hope that this book will provide the reader with ways to implement a variety of group play therapy approaches whatever the platform, medium, or environment.

As stated in the introduction by Mellenthin and Willard, "Group play therapy presents opportunities for the individual child to explore themselves in the context of a social environment and have other children provide feedback, acceptance, and support." It is our hope that you have found gems within these pages that you can incorporate into your play therapy practice to provide powerful and timely services to your clients. May your journey within play therapy continue to be inspirational, exciting, and stimulating.

DOI: 10.4324/9781003094531-102

Index

Printed in the United States
by Baker & Taylor Publisher Services